Eurodrugs

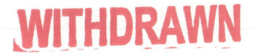

Eurodrugs

Drug use, markets and trafficking in Europe

Vincenzo Ruggiero
Middlesex University

&

Nigel South
University of Essex

UCL
PRESS

First published in 1995 by UCL Press

UCL Press Limited
University College London
Gower Street
London WC1E 6BT

The name of University College London (UCL) is a registered trade mark used by
UCL Press with the consent of the owner.

British Library Cataloguing-in-Publication Data
A CIP catalogue record for this book is available from the British Library.

Library of Congress Cataloging-in-Publication Data

Ruggiero, Vincenzo.
    Eurodrugs: drug use, markets and trafficking in Europe /
Vincenzo Ruggiero and Nigel South.
        p.   cm.
    Includes bibliographical references and index.
    ISBN 1-85728-101-2 (hb). —ISBN 1-85728-102-0 (pb)
    1. Drug traffic—Europe.   2. Drug traffic—Government policy—Europe.
3. Narcotics. Control—Europe.   4. Europe Economic
conditions.   I. South, Nigel.   II. Title.
HV6840.E9R84   1994
363.4'5'094—dc20   94-29846
                                                                        CIP

ISBNs:
1-85728-101-2 HB
1-85728-102-0 PB

Typeset in Plantin
Printed and bound by
Page Bros (Norwich) Ltd., England.

Contents

v

Acknowledgements

First, our grateful thanks to the drug users and dealers who agreed to be interviewed, and to the staff of the library at the Institute for the Study of Drug Dependence, London. Secondly, thanks to Justin Vaughan for taking us on. Thirdly, thanks to Geoff Pearson for some good ideas. Lastly, but of course not least, thanks and love to Cynthia and Lucia and Alison and Daniel.

Nigel South acknowledges the assistance of the Jessie Fuller Bequest Fund, Department of Sociology, University of Essex, for help with research expenses.

VINCENZO RUGGIERO   NIGEL SOUTH
MIDDLESEX UNIVERSITY   UNIVERSITY OF ESSEX
December 1994

1

Introduction

This book is concerned with the topical and important subject of drug use, within the equally topical and important context of the changes occurring within European societies. Its timeliness was recently emphasized by a series of stories on drug use published by *The Independent* newspaper in March 1994. In a major feature on "the European Response" (Doyle 1994: 9), it was argued that "seizures show that the quantity and value of drugs being shipped to the European Union are rising all the time, and the organisations bringing it in are increasingly violent". Unsurprisingly, police and politicians describe such a development "as an ever-escalating threat to European society from the international drugs trade and money-laundering, and organised crime associated with it" (ibid.). Hence, ever-tougher drug control efforts are urged, and from early 1994 a new Europol drugs intelligence unit is in operation to collate information about "top level traffickers". At the same time however, there are increasing numbers of observers across Europe who are willing to support, or at least debate, the possibility of *decriminalizing* some aspects of drug use (Shapiro 1994).

The chapters in this book chart and discuss the growth of drug use in Europe (particularly use of heroin and more recently cocaine) and relate such changes to socio-cultural and political shifts. We also look at this range of responses – differentiated not just by country and culture but also in terms of emphasis, from the tolerance of the Netherlands approach to the more punitive philosophy of other countries. Common agreement that drug-related crime and HIV/AIDS are serious problems has not been accompanied by common implementation of policy or practice. Yet, more than ever before, an adequate understanding of drug use in any one European country demands appreciation of developments elsewhere in Europe. And, of course, what we mean by "Europe" has itself changed dramatically in recent years, with quite specific and important implications for patterns of drug use and international trafficking. As eastern Europe opens up and internal trade barriers fall, drug distribution and markets benefit just as much as (indeed, perhaps more than) legal enterprises. Furthermore, analysis of drug markets must acknowledge that the expansion of trading opportunities in a prosperous economic area such as Europe, facilitates not only legitimate but also illegal transactions with entrepreneurs in countries that produce plant drugs, where domestic economies generally have a desperate need to pull in western currency.

In this chapter, we shall sketch out past approaches in the criminological study of drug use, markets and trafficking and outline our own perspective; discuss our aims and methods; and finally, offer five propositions or hypotheses that are addressed in the course of the book.

Drugs and criminology

From the 19th century to the 1950s, positivist criminology was concerned to identify forms of pathology among drug users. In the critical reaction to this school which developed from the 1960s on, studies principally focused on the institutional responses (law, policy, media etc.) to drug use. This and societal disapproval were argued to be the real forces that shape the nature of the drug problem. For many of the "new deviancy theorists" of the 1960s and 1970s, what was at stake was an important cultural and political principle: legislation should not intrude in matters of personal choice or "victimless crimes". When state and law intervene in such cases, they simply exacerbate the "problem" if one exists, or create one if it does not. The concept of "deviancy amplification" was central to such a perspective (Young 1971a,b).

In the 1980s, analysis of drug use and users shifted attention. Drug problems were no longer seen as simply the result of excessive institutional and public reaction to drugs; rather drug use became a symbol and symptom of deeper and more complex social problems, which are compounded by the cumulative effects of experiences such as unemployment, marginalization, general vulnerability and so on. This shift of analysis was a momentous one. However, our perspective here tries to avoid the extremes of these various positions – the polarity of individual pathology vs. social construction and the uneasy balancing of individual marginalization and social determinism. We identify two key propositions which, we hope, will help us to do this and also guide the reader through the following chapters.

A market approach

First, our primary orientation is to regard illicit drugs simply as commodities. These commodities shape and are shaped by demand and supply, exchange and consumption. In order to pre-empt accusations of "vulgar materialism", "simple economism" etc., we should emphasize that we do not concentrate only on the material conditions in which these commodities are produced, distributed and consumed. We also assume that drug use is embedded in socio-cultural contexts which change in time and space. This assumption will inevitably lead us to pay attention to both micro and macro structural influences on drug use, cultures and markets.

To give one example of how drugs can be seen as undergoing a process of "commodification", we can cite the practice of "labelling" doses, wraps or deals. This has been a long established marketing strategy in New York and other North American cities (Inciardi 1986) and has been familiar in Europe in relation to batches of LSD and ecstasy. Cannabis and heroin have also been reported for sale in London under "brand names" (Hyder 1993). This process simply involves packaging drugs in distinctive coloured paper and attaching a similarly distinctive commercial name that will help the consumers identify their favoured product. The marketing aim is that users become accustomed to using one "variety", less on the basis of chemical composition than its commercial identity. As with designer-label clothes, users may demand "brand names" (Goldstein et al. 1984, Inciardi 1986). There are two points to note here: first, illegal markets are unstable and lack the solid infrastructure of legitimate sales operations – e.g. stores and products that can be found in the market place day after day. Without this stability and continuity then "brand loyalties" will be fragile and easily displaced. Secondly, as many of the street drug "brand names" suggest, drug markets reproduce (and may amplify) the inequalities, sexism and prejudices of the wider society. We shall return to these general points.

Our second orientating perspective is that we suggest an interpretation of the illegal activities associated with drug use and distribution as *work*. This perspective is inspired by a substantial body of criminological analysis to which we are indebted. Letkenmann (1973: 159) has usefully summarized this perspective in the following terms:

> I have shown how such concepts as specialization, professionalism, apprenticeship, and work satisfaction may help us understand criminal behavior. . . . The work perspective draws attention to the various skills and abilities required of persons in various conventional work roles. The presence or absence of specialized skills is commonly used to explain wage differentials and work satisfaction. I have argued that a recognition of the various skills required in criminal activity may, likewise, help explain variations in status and work satisfaction among criminals.

This emphasis upon characteristics such as "specialization", "skills" and "professionalism", is central to the analysis presented here.

Mack (1964) utilized a similar perspective when studying a number of criminal activities. The dimension of "work" was incorporated in his definition of the "full-time miscreant". He remarked:

> criminality is a normal aspect of the social structure, a permanent feature of any complex society, an ongoing social activity like the practice of medicine or police work or university teaching or stevedoring. It is sustained, like these other activities, by a sub-culture of people and groups most of whom are tolerably well-adjusted to their sub-culture

and most of whose leaders are not only socially and personally competent but are also exceptionally able individuals (ibid.: 52).

A similar approach was adopted by Einstadter (1969) and Shover (1973) in their studies of, respectively, the social organization of armed robbery, and burglary. Both authors identified the salient "occupational" aspects of the two crimes and their evolution, in terms of techniques and occupational culture, which were regarded as the result of changes in the economy on the one hand, and in the nature of security protection services and devices on the other (South 1988). Similarly, McIntosh (1971: 98) suggested that criminals can be studied like any other occupational group. When investigating the organization of thieving, she stressed that, "Professional criminals follow the rules and customs of their work much as other workers do". She also argued that criminologists should not only study why people take up criminal occupations, "but also how the occupational tasks are divided up and interrelated, how working groups and occupational communities with hierarchies of status and of authority are formed, and what the relations between these groups and communities and other groups are like" (ibid.).

The authors referred to above are but a few of those whose contributions are central to the perspective of the present book. The development of our arguments also draws on work that is more specifically concerned with illicit drugs and drug-related occupations. Among these, we must, in particular, mention Preble & Casey (1969), whose pioneering work described the life and activities of lower-class heroin users in New York City in the context of their street environment. In addition, Agar's (1973) study of heroin users was based on extensive contact and offered a description of the major events of the users' occupational culture (hustling, copping and getting-off). Agar conducted his study in an institutional setting and other authors have tried to overcome the problems this poses by contacting active members of the drug economy who were unknown to official agencies. Hughes et al. (1971), for example, used field-workers who were assigned to a heroin distribution site or "copping area" in a Chicago neighbourhood. During a year of observation, the field team determined that the majority of the subjects contacted could be described as playing one of the following rôles: big dealer, street dealer, part-time dealer, bag follower, tout, hustler, and worker. This descriptive approach and interest in the division of labour in drug markets, also inform our study.

In the 1980s, a more detailed, ethnographic approach was fruitfully adopted by Adler (1985) in her study of an upper-level drug dealing and smuggling community in California. Adler found that drug dealers and smugglers did not abandon conventional society and enter an underworld of deviance because their legitimate opportunities were blocked. Their entry into the illicit drug economy was influenced by various factors and Lewis (1993) finds Adler's analysis broadly translatable to the European context. At the other end of the distribution hierarchy, Hanson et al. (1985: 1) studied the inner-city heroin milieu in Chicago, New York, Washington, DC, and Philadelphia. Their book relied on the users' own words "to describe lives that revolve around the use of heroin – lifestyles in which a 'jones' (heroin habit) is a constant companion . . .".

Coming to more recent influences. First, we must mention the work of Peter Reuter. His early work on *Disorganised crime* (1983) obviously influences our critique of monopolistic models of criminal organization. More recently, Reuter et al. (1990) have described the rôle of street drug-selling in the economic life of young males in Washington, DC. This study estimated the number of persons involved in drug supply at this level and described their social characteristics. What Reuter et al. found disturbing from their analysis, was the relatively high *employment* rate among dealers. In their view, this could be interpreted in the following way: "drug dealing is an underground version of 'moonlighting' – it provides a high-paying supplement to regular employment but cannot be converted into the primary job" (ibid.: ix). As a consequence, the authors argue, job creation *per se* may do little to reduce willingness to participate in drug markets (we develop a similar argument below). In other words, drug dealing may provide illegal "occasional work" for urban males seeking supplementary income, it need not be their principal occupation: "in particular, drug dealing may provide the kinds of employment opportunities, in terms of working infrequent hours, that college students derive from waiting tables in restaurants" (ibid.: 77). Such evidence and argument supports the kind of labour market analysis that we develop here.

We would also draw attention to Davis's (1992) account of the political economy of crack in Los Angeles, where the author remarks: "if the estimate of 10,000 gang members making their livelihood from the drug trade is anywhere near correct, then crack really is the employer of last resort in the ghetto's devastated Eastside – the equivalent of several large auto plants or several hundred MacDonalds" (ibid.: 314). In addition, we have found recent ethnographic work on drugs economies in the USA, of interest. For example, Williams's (1989; 1992) research on the occupational rôles within the crack economy and crack houses in New York; and similarly work by Bourgois (1989) and Hamid (1990). A mention is also due to Padilla's (1992) study of gangs as enterprises, where the author considers gang-sponsored illegal activities, such as drug dealing, in occupational terms, and regards the "job of the drug dealer as being like other conventional work" (ibid.: 4). In England, Pearson's work in the North and in the London region, on socioeconomic aspects of the drug users' life should also be noted (e.g. 1987a,b, Mirza et al. 1991). Finally, of course, we also draw upon our own past work and acknowledge the influence of colleagues and collaborators (Ruggiero 1986, Ruggiero & Vass 1992, Dorn & South 1990, Dorn et al. 1992).

A comparative perspective on drugs in Europe

This book draws upon the literature noted above and, of course, much more. Indeed, we hope that the substantial bibliography will be a useful resource for others. But this is only the starting point for our attempt to develop a broader *European* perspective. Our aim is to provide a comparative account of illegal drug use, markets and trafficking in Europe – a perspective that is often absent in the English language literature. We are aware that this situation is changing, of course. Studies have begun to examine some aspects of the development of drug related crime, enforcement and legislation in Europe (Albrecht & van Kalmthout 1989, Dorn & South 1991a, Flood 1991, Savona et al. 1994), yet work which offers a comparative perspective is still rare, and in relation to studies of drug markets and drug users, it is rarer still. The chapters that follow draw upon research material from across Europe, and describe the changes which have taken place in the values and activities of those participating in illegal drug markets through the 1970s, 1980s and into the 1990s.

We first provide a European framework. In Chapters 2 and 3, we review drug use, cultures, markets and trafficking in Europe. We also briefly consider some matters of policy, such as treatment approaches and control issues, concluding Chapter 3 with a discussion of the prospects for liberalization of drug use laws in Europe. In Chapters 4 and 5, we focus on two countries in particular, Britain and Italy, which offer interesting comparisons as "case studies". More specifically, the case studies and original research concentrate on two areas within these countries: Greater London and the industrial area of Turin and Piedmont in the North West of Italy.

Obviously, we focus on these because they are our "home" countries, but even if this was not the case there are excellent grounds for taking these areas as case studies. First, they reflect particularly interesting examples of the development and histories of drug cultures and markets. Secondly, they are countries which offer well established traditions of drug research with a substantial body of epidemiological, descriptive and analytical studies. Thirdly, trends in these two countries may be clearer than in some others, and although cultures and histories will obviously differ between these and in relation to other countries, nonetheless such trends may suggest policy conclusions which have a wider applicability (see Hartnoll 1986: 71). Fourthly, the two case studies provide material which suggest the need for a re-discussion and re-definition of "organized crime". Criminologically, Italy and Britain have long been regarded as countries which present two incomparable crime patterns; the former being characterized by long-established, structured and highly organized criminal activities, the latter by more recent, less developed forms of criminal organization and a high incidence of diffuse, opportunistic, "street level" criminality. However, the significance of the drug economy in both contexts makes a comparison between the two countries appropriate. In terms of moves towards a more unified Europe, the removal of border controls, growth of East–West trade and general trends towards globalized markets, examination of the broader European context is both urgent and vital (Interpol 1990, Flood 1991).

We shall assess our findings in Chapter 6.

A note on methods and respondents

We adopt here a "case study" method, with the aims of providing qualitative description of specific contexts and contours of drug related activity, and the hope that this method facilitates comparison. We are cautious about generalizing from these cases and aware of the limitations of this approach. As our earlier review of significant literature suggests, we seek to avoid at least one pitfall of this method by developing our arguments in ways which also draw upon data and theories from beyond our specific findings (Platt 1993: 12).

The core material for the two case studies derives from work carried out by both authors in Greater London and SE England, between 1985 and 1993, and by Ruggiero in Italy, throughout the 1980s and into the 1990s. In addition, the book is based on extensive reading of relevant European and international literature – both academic and official; plus unpublished reports, briefings and agency materials. For the two case study countries interviews were conducted with ex- and current users, distributors, social workers, drug street agency staff, police and probation officers, and Customs and Excise staff. In Italy, traffickers and distributors with experience of dealing in up to half a kilo of heroin (and other drugs) were also interviewed. In Greater London, we have made use of field-work notes and interview transcripts for contacts with over 100 drug users, ex-users and user-dealers; plus over 25 interviews with police, probation and social work staff. In addition, Ruggiero's recent case study of Lambeth (Ruggiero 1993a) provided over 50 interviews with drug workers, users, dealers, residents, police etc. and his work in Turin has now involved "snowballing" through several waves of heroin users, producing numerous interviews.

Themes of the book

This book is guided by a set of themes which form hypothetical propositions. They are addressed throughout the following chapters and re-assessed in Chapter 6. These propositions are "idealized" and generated from the views of other writers and broader popular assumptions – we did not expect them all to be proved "true".

These propositions are:

1) Drugs have become key commodities within the traditional criminal underworld and this has generated an impulse towards more structured forms of criminality, and has enhanced the organizational character of some criminal activities. In this process, a tendency may be observed whereby "diffuse" crime and so-called opportunistic crime may end up being linked with illegal activities carried out on a larger scale.

2) In the activities connected to drug distribution, we may observe monopolistic tendencies in permanent conflict with strong counter-tendencies of a competitive nature that fragment the market.

3) The explosion of availability of illegal drugs during the 1980s (undiminished in the 1990s) can be seen as impacting upon certain forms of criminal enterprise, which we tentatively describe as "crime in association" and "crime in organization". These definitions allude to two different modes of criminal "work" and two respective models of organization and structure. A horizontal structure prevails in the former, a vertical one in the latter. "Crime in association" implies individual entrepreneuriality in a non-hierarchical structure. Here, the division of labour is technical not social, in the sense that tasks are allocated on the basis of skills not of social rôles or status. "Crime in organization" implies an industrial or corporate style structure, whereby "criminal labour" is exchanged for a salary (paid in various forms). In classical terms, the division of labour in this case is of a social nature. We hypothesize that the development of drug economies may favour a tendential shift from the former towards the latter type of structure. We shall elaborate on these "types" later.

4) Relatedly, there may be shifts occurring in relation to "types" of criminal activity. Borrowing terms from the sociology of work, we hypothesize that "professional" criminals of a traditional skilled type may now – as with the de-skilling of legitimate, traditional occupations – be partly replaced by "mass" criminals ("mass workers") working in a *chain* of production and distribution. The definition of "mass worker" is well known within the European political science and sociological tradition. This describes the Fordist-type industrial worker

who contributed to the productive boom in countries such as France, Germany and Italy. The classic examples of "mass workers" have been Arabs employed by Renault in France, Turks working for Volkswagen in Germany and the South Italians employed by Fiat and other industries in Northern Italy. Such industrial workers, who had only recently left their rural environment, have been described as excluded from the traditional route through apprenticeship to skilled labour and a strong identification with their new work. Unlike their professional counterparts, they therefore have no feeling of satisfaction in relation to their job, which is repetitive and alienating. Their tasks are limited and their knowledge of the productive cycle in which they are engaged is negligible. Our definition of the "mass" criminal is intended to echo these sociological characteristics, and apply it to a section of "labourers" who are employed within the drug economy. In other words, we hypothesize that a process is underway whereby many individuals engaged in drug use and distribution will become more and more involved in the criminal drug economy. However, in the criminal activities they undertake, they will increasingly lack specific skills, the benefit of a "traditional apprenticeship" (or equivalent experience), and/or specialist knowledge concerning the overall cycle of enterprise in which they participate.

5) Finally and crucially, drug cultures and markets have undergone changes which demand a re-appraisal of the conventional sociological theory usually employed for their interpretation. We refer here to subcultural and anomie perspectives, which are still dominant in discussions of drug use and dealing. But do the insights and claims of theories from the 1930s, 1940s, 1950s and 1960s still stand? Given that their development and application was principally in the context of North American society, are they in need of modification to explain drug use and markets in Europe, at the end of the 20th century? In Chapter 6 a critique of these perspectives is offered.

11

2

Drug use in Europe: patterns, cultures and policies

This book is concerned with markets, cultures, structures and networks, in which illegal drugs feature as commodities. We are also concerned with drug users, dealers and entrepreneurial others who play various rôles in these social and economic structures. In Chapters 4 and 5, below, we detail case studies of London and of Turin. In this and the following chapter we shall offer a broader picture of patterns of drug use, markets, crime, trafficking and controls across Europe. We cannot, however, treat each country entirely fairly and equally. We are faced with limitations in terms of available information, available time and available space! We can, however, present data and descriptions that should give the reader a better picture of the broad canvas of European drug use, markets and cultures than has been available up to now and our referencing of other studies will enable researchers to pursue their own specific interests further. In our unequal allocation of space and attention here, we present more information on some countries than others. Hence, these chapters provide more detailed accounts of the situation in our case study countries, Britain and Italy, as well as two other countries with differing but well known and significant drug problem histories – the Netherlands in western Europe and Poland in eastern Europe. We shall also describe developments in most other major European countries but in less detail.

Epidemiological overviews

Few studies offer much of an overview of patterns of drug use in Europe or of the interconnectedness of policy development, enforcement co-operation (and competition), political accord or research co-ordination. There are some exceptions, however, and we hope that we draw on most here. Regarding epidemiology, Hartnoll (1989: 44) offers a succinct picture of heroin availability and use across Europe up to the late 1980s:

> During the late 1960s and early 1970s, there was evidence of increased use in some of the more northern European countries, including Britain, the Netherlands, Germany, Denmark, and France. However, it was not until the second half of the 1970s that the supply and use of heroin escalated rapidly across Europe, including countries such as Italy, Spain, Ireland, Switzerland, Austria and Greece that had little prior experience of illicit heroin.

Acknowledging that there were (and are) "no accurate estimates", Hartnoll suggested that by the late 1980s, the number of addicts in Europe may have been over half a million.

Regarding cocaine, Lewis (1989: 48–49) provides an overview of conditions affecting the European market from the 1970s on:

> A relative abundance at source contributed to the growth of the European market, although cocaine remains the most expensive stimulant available. There was a period of gradual, but sustained, increases in price and production in South America during the 1970s. This was followed by sharp price fluctuations between 1980 and 1985 that resulted from alternate gluts and shortages in supply in the classic boom-and-bust cycle of many other tropical products. Characteristically, there was a time lag as the effects passed along the supply chain, fluctuations tending to be less extreme the closer one came to the centres of consumption. However, the glut of 1983–4, when kilos could be purchased in Columbia for one-quarter of their 1982 price, impacted upon the farthest reaches of the European

retail market where gram prices fell on occasions by as much as forty per cent.

However, a recent review of "the spread of cocaine in Europe" (Barrio-Anta 1991) notes that "in spite of the sharp increase in supply over recent years, it has been impossible to ascertain an increase in cocaine-related problems. . . . It is possible that in the coming years there will be an increase in cocaine-related problems; although perhaps not such a spectacular one as some people have predicted." (ibid.: 146)

In terms of drug distribution generally, Lewis (1989: 50–51) argues that trafficking groups in producer countries and those operating as cross-border multinational enterprises, see Europe as one large "continental market", rather than divided into individual countries. We shall examine methods and patterns of trafficking in the next chapter.

In the latter part of the 1970s, use of volatile solvents (glue, butane etc.) increased in parts of the United Kingdom, France and Germany, particularly among youths of 12–16 years old. Related deaths caused considerable alarm in these countries (Hartnoll 1986: 69). Since the 1970s, use of barbiturates seems to have declined in Germany, UK and Ireland, following changes in prescribing practice and related to the rising popularity of heroin. LSD use generally fell in European countries in the late 1970s and early 1980s but countries such as the UK, the Netherlands, France and Spain have recently seen a resurgence of use of this and other psychedelic drugs such as MDMA (ecstasy) related to, first, Acid House, and then Rave music/dance culture (Redhead 1993). Hartnoll also provides a rough assessment of variation among the social characteristics of drug users across Europe.

It will be obvious that drug use and drug problems will be unevenly spread and differentiated across Europe and, therefore, future work might profitably adapt and apply the three levels of analysis which Pearson & Gilman (1994: 105) describe as "macro-diffusion", "urban clustering" and "micro-diffusion":

At the broadest level, we can identify processes of "macro-diffusion" which involve the diffusion of drug practices across time and between different regions. This process was well exemplified by the work of Hunt & Chambers (1976) which examined the North American heroin epidemics from the mid-1960s to the mid-1970s. In their study the geographical distance between towns and cities, together with the ease of communication routes between regions, proved to be a major determinant of the macro-diffusion of drug habits . . .

At the other end of the spectrum, "micro-diffusion" is the means by which drugs and drug practices move within friendship networks within a locality. People are invariably first introduced to drug practices by friends, rather than "pushers" . . . The spread of drug habits at this level will be encouraged or inhibited, not by environmental factors such as geographical distance and terrain, but by local sub-cultural preferences.

Our case study chapters provide various examples of both polar types of "drug use diffusion". The third level of analysis distinguished by Pearson & Gilman, falls between these two poles and is termed "urban clustering" "reflecting the ways in which some neighbourhoods (and not others) become the sites of concentration of drug problems in any given town or city." Pearson & Gilman suggest that such locations

will invariably be areas of high social deprivation. This is perhaps the most complex level of analysis and involves social processes such as the mechanism of the housing market, the workings of the "irregular economy" and the exchange of illicit goods and services, and lifestyles associated with long-term unemployment.

We shall discuss the issues of social deprivation, marginality and drug use later in this chapter, and pay particular attention to the interactions between licit and illicit markets for labour and commodities in our two case study chapters.

In terms of macro-developments, Wever (1992: 177) attempts a swift but neat overview of European and wider global trends:

Illicit opium production in south-east Asia doubled in

1989 and stabilised on that level in 1990. Heroin trafficking from China increased, whilst trafficking and drug use in the Thailand and Malaysia region stabilised. The production of opium in large parts of Laos and Myanmar (Burma) is completely out of government control . . . In some parts of south Asia, such as Bangladesh and India, drug use is on the rise, particularly on trafficking routes. Poppy production in the Near and Middle East, especially in Pakistan, Afghanistan, Iran – despite tough governmental measures – and Lebanon continues . . .

The current political and economic changes in several central and eastern European countries has resulted in a substantial increase in the movement of people and goods, including illicit drugs. In the former Soviet Union the number of drug users has doubled during the last five years. The seizure figures for heroin and cocaine in western Europe continue to rise steadily. It appears that cocaine use is spreading. Among drug addicts heroin is still the major drug of choice, although the number of users seems to have stabilised and the average age has risen. On the other hand, in some European countries, the level of HIV infection among intravenous drug users is extremely high.

Case study countries:

Britain: England

Heroin history: use, cultures, availability and policy
In Britain, cannabis remains the most popular illegal drug in use, yet social concern, policy debate and research interest have, primarily, focused on *heroin*. (Recent comprehensive analyses and discussions of data on trends in drug use and availability are to be found in ISDD/Ashton 1993 and Sutton & Maynard 1992; we briefly discuss use of other drugs in Britain below. For more detailed descriptions of the history of patterns of use, availability and control in Britain see Pearson 1990, South 1994).

During the 19th century opiates were widely available throughout Europe and North America as medicines, tonics and childrens' "quietners" (Berridge & Edwards 1981, Musto 1973). Recreational and intoxicant use was known in certain industrial, dockside and farming regions, and had some popularity in limited middle-class and bohemian circles. However, in the latter part of the century and into the early decades of the next, there were increasing pressures for, and finally implementation of, controls over the availability of opiates, and also cocaine (Berridge & Edwards 1981, Kohn 1992). Moral opposition grew towards Britain's deep involvement in the international opium trade and new medical discourses contributed to a change in perception of such narcotic use – from an indulgence that could be tolerated to a problem or mania, classifiable and treatable by the intervention of science. In the early years of the First World War, concerns were aroused that threats to the security of the nation and the efficiency of the troops were posed by cocaine use and prostitution. Press and public were fascinated by such a suggestion and in 1916 Home Office officials seized the opportunity to use emergency war legislation as a means of introducing regulations over the supply of cocaine and opium (Defence of the Realm Act, regulation 40B, Berridge 1978, Kohn 1992). Between the end of the war and the mid to late 1920s, various forms of drug use in Britain had a degree of visibility and sensation attached to them that had far less to do with their actual prevalence than their treatment in the press and cinema of the day (Kohn 1992). In reality, opiate and cocaine users were to be found in diminishing numbers under treatment by a doctor, in the opium dens of Limehouse or among the cocaine "fast set" of the West End. Even as the famous Rolleston Committee deliberated on the future of addiction policy in Britain and presented its report in 1926, drug use as a problem of any magnitude or significance was fading away. For the period between the 1930s and the late 1950s, the so-called "British system", bequeathed by Rolleston, is frequently portrayed as having been the successful bulwark against drug problems that might otherwise have developed as they did in the United States. In fact, as Downes (1977: 89) observes, this "system" represented "little more than masterly inactivity in the face of what was an almost nonexistent addiction problem."

As Lart (1992: 118) neatly summarizes:

Between the Rolleston report of 1926 and the second Brain

report of 1965, what has been known as the "British system" of treating addiction dominated the field ... in the United Kingdom. The basis of this was that any medical practitioner was permitted to use his or her own professional judgement in the decision to prescribe what were known as addictive drugs, in the treatment of a person believed to be addicted to those drugs.

During this period, the definition of addiction and the image of the drug user changed dramatically, from that of an individualised pathology affecting unfortunates, to a socially infectious condition, needing to be controlled.

The issue of control moved to centre stage because of the emergence of *a market* in illicit drugs, particularly heroin, between the early to mid 1960s, when one grain (64 mg.) could be purchased for £1 (Stimson & Oppenheimer 1982). Up until 1968 this market offered 100 per cent pure heroin, which could be legally obtained with a medical prescription. Prescribed pharmaceutical heroin, therefore, fed a "grey market" – suspended between legality and incomplete criminalization (Lewis et al. 1985).

The so-called "British System" (Whynes & Bean 1991), initially permitting maintenance of addicts on pure heroin, attracted a significant number of users from Canada and the USA. These early "drug tourists" found that not only could they obtain heroin at reasonable prices, but also consume it in comparatively low risk conditions. Between 1961 and 1968 the number of heroin addicts notified to the Home Office increased from around 50 to 1000 (Glass 1982). Early signs of an increase had, in fact, been discernible at the end of the 1950s, but at the time that the 1958 Brain Committee was preparing its report (Interdepartmental Committee on Drug Addiction 1961), the 1961 statistics were still unavailable. Hence the Committee recognized some concern about increased availability of cannabis and heroin but concluded that supply was really quite negligible. Little amendment to policy and practice was needed! The 1961 addict statistics, however, showed that change was occurring, the number of addicts was rising and, while modest, the rise continued (Mott 1991:78–9, Lart 1992: 122). The Brain Committee was reconvened in 1964 and its report of the following year was to have a major impact on the development of British drug control and treatment (Lart 1992: 123–4, Stimson & Oppenheimer 1982).

Among the users of pharmaceutical heroin during the 1960s, many were part of the new youth cultures and bohemias of music and art. Others, only marginally involved in the London art scene, also scored in this new market. Cannabis and LSD homologously fitted with the style, values and music of the counterculture (Auld 1981, Willis 1978), while other youth cultures adopted other drug use patterns, such as the Mods employment of amphetamine to keep going through the weekend (Cohen 1972).

From 1968 the authority to prescribe heroin and cocaine was limited by new regulations to a relatively small number of specialists, principally psychiatrists. New Drug Dependency Units were established in and around London where the drug problem was reckoned to be, and adopted the North American model of prescribing methadone as a substitute for heroin. In 1970 pharmaceutical heroin was only prescribed to 10 per cent of the registered habitual users and methadone to 51 per cent (Brecher 1972). In 1975 the two quota were respectively 4.5 per cent and 67 per cent (Ray 1978).

Although modest, the spread of heroin use in the 1960s had aroused official concern and the dominant explanation, quickly accepted, was that certain doctors were prescribing with unprofessional laxity (Leech 1991, Mott 1991, Lart 1992). The degree of this casualness is still a controversial subject, however. According to one general practitioner with memories of this period:

> Both the media and the government grossly exaggerated the figures. Rumours went that some doctors in the West End would prescribe something like a thousand doses in one go. Things were not exactly so: some doctors were simply more humane than others, they understood that the youths they were facing had serious problems and just tried to help them. The quantity prescribed was that which the patient needed, or perhaps that which the doctor thought the patient needed. (Interview)

The discussion regarding the responsibilities of practitioners has continued – through the early 1980s, when the *British Medical Jour-*

nal hosted contributions that were pro or con the maintenance model, and later in the decade when the upsurge in heroin use stimulated more debate about prescribing (Ashton 1986a,b), up to today, when some Government ministers are questioning the principles of maintenance prescribing and harm minimization (Druglink 1993: 5). Nonetheless some consensus produced general criteria for maintenance prescribing: in order to prevent users from resorting to the illegal market, the quantity of heroin prescribed would not be reduced by too much, but nor would prescribing be too high, thereby seeking to avoid a surplus feeding the grey market (Edwards 1978).

Accusations of fraud or private interest, implicit or explicit, overshadowed some doctors for years, often based on the assumption that their prescribing practice was cynically abused simply to provide them with increased income (Bewley & Ghodse 1983). In 1981, an Association of Independent Doctors was formed with the aim of responding to such criticism. Their argument was that independent doctors were not creating problems but rather that they were doing much to contain them by minimizing the need for addicts to turn to property crime (Dally 1983). Such vituperation continued despite the fact that by the late 1970s and early 1980s, a new generation of users had already largely altered the social profile of heroin use along with the characteristics of the market in Britain (Dally 1990).

Between 1973 and 1977 official notification of new narcotic users numbered 4607 (Giggs 1991: 153). Growth of opioid use was relatively limited but steady; use was often combined with barbiturate-type drugs, and the scene remained largely concentrated around London. However, once again changes were occurring. According to one ex-user interviewed:

> By the mid-1970s those who bought heroin were no longer the old junkies who were well known to their doctors, and got the stuff either from a friendly chemist or from the Drug Dependence Units. New users came in. These were young people who had no intention of becoming officially registered as heroin users and preferred to buy Iranian, Chinese or Thai stuff, illegally imported, which was already available.

It could be suggested that many of the new users resorted to the illicit market because they felt that an "alternative" arena would provide them with a more attractive identity – one which was beating the system. Seeing a doctor can entail disempowerment and submission to the expectations of the "sick rôle" (Turner 1987). It involves delegation of authority to someone else, "an expert", over one's own health and choice. Involvement in the illicit market may be a means of retaining a sense of empowered identity and control.

However, among our respondents, this hypothesis was only partly accepted. Rather, it was argued that the growth of the illicit market was the direct consequence of new legislation and restrictions limiting the power of doctors to prescribe. Thus, while the official view is that the growth of an illicit heroin market was caused by unrestricted prescribing by independent, private doctors, several of our respondents with knowledge of this period argued the opposite, i.e. that the restrictions on prescribing caused the growth of the illicit market. Thus, the spread of illegal heroin is attributed by these respondents to the decline of the maintenance model and the rôle that "independent" prescribers had played within it. No doubt the dynamics of market growth can be argued to owe something to both these "causes" (see Leech 1991: 54). The latter view also places prescribers of the period in a rather saintly position: far from pursuing personal advantage, the generosity of such doctors was described as a mixture of naïvete, unfamiliarity with how drugs might be used illicitly and their effects, and a degree of countercultural sympathy. One ex-user, now a drug worker, suggested:

> The doctors who prescribed more were highly motivated in the ideological sense. Some of them were culturally very close to the users and were part of that "alternative" world of the 1960s. Well known to drug users, they would behave like friends with their clients and in fact they shared the same subculture with them. To these doctors, drugs constituted a challenge against the official society and a political and cultural threat to official values such as productivity, sobriety, efficiency. These doctors, if unwittingly, contributed to a certain extent to the spread of heroin in Britain.

This may be an atypical and unorthodox interpretation of the politics of prescribing during the 1960s and 1970s, but should be taken seriously precisely for running counter to the conventional and standard histories.

In the next chapter we shall consider how this relatively small-scale and domestic heroin scene of the 1970s was transformed by international developments and the widespread availability, from the end of that decade, of a "new" form of smokeable heroin.

Other drugs

Despite the early concerns about cocaine use which had arisen during World War One and the early 1920s (Berridge 1978, 1979, Kohn 1992, Spear & Mott 1992), cocaine has not typically been in high demand in Britain or the rest of Europe. Usually regarded as a "champagne drug", it has been expensive and generally had more of an association with American drug culture. As a stimulant drug suitable for snorting or injecting, amphetamine has generally proved to be far more popular. However, in the early 1970s, demand and availability saw increased use of cocaine among recreational users. Lewis (1989: 41) describes the London market for cocaine at this time:

> The interpenetration of the fashion, music and entertainment industries in the United Kingdom, and the cultural influence of North America contributed to the increased acceptability of cocaine.
>
> ... Formerly, cocaine had been limited to small circles of the bohemian rich and a growing population of heroin addicts. Most drug users restricted themselves to cannabis, LSD and pharmaceutical amphetamine preparations. Prior to 1968 cocaine, like heroin, could be prescribed by any doctor for the treatment of an addictive condition. Hence, most cocaine originated in or was diverted from legitimate pharmaceutical sources. By historical coincidence, recreational cocaine use began to expand in London at the very time that specialist physicians had effectively ceased to prescribe the drug in the treatment of addiction.

Cocaine is usually taken by nasal ingestion, though some users may inject, and a few may "freebase", smoking the drug. Use cuts across all social classes although the drug remains relatively expensive and retains an association with elites and glamour. Its use in Britain has not become as widespread as often predicted – nor has there been an overwhelming flood of crack on the streets. Enforcement and independent reports (Miles 1993, Bean & Pearson 1992, Dean 1991, Dean et al. 1992, Shapiro 1989, 1991, 1993) agree that in certain areas Britain is seeing modest to sizeable local markets in crack developing, but the high profile "crack attack" panic promoted in the late 1980s by commentators from the USA and media coverage has not yet seen any justification (Shapiro, ibid.). Parts of south London have repeatedly been identified as areas of cocaine/ crack availability, but between 1987 and 1989 Strang et al. (1990) found that only four out of 425 clients at a local drug service identified cocaine as their main problem drug. However, other data did indicate an increase in numbers of cocaine users among new clients to some services, with up to three-quarters smoking the drug. Most were white, with one-quarter from ethnic minority groups.

Obviously, the picture is still unclear. Users reporting cocaine addiction to drug agencies may actually be using crack, and vice versa; some heroin users in our study occasionally tried cocaine because it "gives [them] the buzz"; while some heavy cocaine and crack users start using heroin for its depressant effects: "I see a lot of people using cocaine and as a result they often start using heroin. Heroin will deal with the paranoia, the anxiety, the tension caused by cocaine. But they deny they use heroin: publicly they only use cocaine!" (user-dealer).

We shall explore the changing rôle of cocaine/crack in the London and UK drugs economy further in Chapter 4.

Britain: Scotland

Reports from Glasgow (Ditton & Speirits 1981) were among the first to draw attention to the dramatic expansion of heroin use occurring at the end of the 1970s and beginning of the 1980s. As Pearson (1991: 185) records, "at first this had appeared to be an isolated occurrence and even led to some controversy among drug specialists in Scotland that a 'moral panic' was being fuelled unnecessarily. However, subsequent research confirmed that not only was Glasgow a major site of heroin misuse, but also that epidemic forms of misuse had developed in other parts of Scotland such as Edinburgh (Haw 1985, Ditton & Taylor 1987, McKeganey & Boddy 1987, Morrison 1988)". More recently, a snowball-study of 135 regular drug users in Edinburgh and Ayr has provided important findings about new preferences for multiple drug use, found to be common among both injecting and non-injecting users, with injectors increasingly using licit, prescribed drugs such as temazepam (a "sleeping pill") and buprenorphine (an opioid). Difficulties in obtaining heroin have not, therefore, reduced injecting behaviours (Morrison 1989). A study of "use of buprenorphine and temazepam by drug injectors" in Glasgow (Lavelle et al. 1991) found a similar trend (ISDD/Ashton 1993: 44).

Problem drug use in Scotland has received much publicity and considerable research attention in relation to crime and health issues (notably HIV/AIDS but also alcohol use) (Hammersley et al. 1989, 1990, Morrison 1991, 1992). However, there are some patterns of drug use which seem relatively unproblematic. The Scottish Cocaine Research Group have published descriptions of 92 cocaine users for whom neither chronic dependence nor major associated problems have developed (Ditton et al. 1991). Drawn from a wide range of contacts and agencies around Glasgow and Edinburgh, these users fit "neither the stereotype of the wealthy cocaine snorter nor that of the delinquent crack smoker. They reside instead on the fringe of middle-class respectability, having some employment, some money, some other drugs, some problems, but never very much of anything" (ibid.: 275; see also Cohen 1989).

Scotland has had a markedly worse experience with drug related HIV and cases of AIDS (albeit with local variation) than England and Wales. Edinburgh in particular, reaped the sad consequences of policies opposing maintenance prescribing and syringe exchanges and rates of HIV infection reached over 50 per cent among intravenous drug users in the city by the mid 1980s (Robertson et al. 1986). In Glasgow, with more liberal policies in place, HIV infection in the same period was less than 5 per cent (Follett et al. 1986). As Morrison (1992: 50) observes, "multiple deprivation undermines a lot of positive work being done in Edinburgh (and elsewhere in Scotland). This is a political problem which requires tackling at the grass roots level. What is needed is a 'voice' to defend the rights of people with HIV and, equally those who care for them."

Italy

Italy has only developed drug problems related to the use of *illegal drugs* relatively recently. During the early 1970s the illicit use of drugs was associated with the growth of youth countercultures and only rarely regarded as symptomatic of a broader social problem. Drug abuse was presented as a purely individual expression of malaise and most frequently its origin was traced to affluence. This explanation stood out significantly in a study of the public image of drug abuse in national daily newspapers (Blumir et al. 1975). None of the papers examined hinted at quasi-sociological explanations for use, such as links between drug abuse and marginalization. In discussion of drug trafficking and distribution, journalistic emphasis was placed almost entirely upon the street dealers and couriers. Description concentrated on drug users in the upper middle-classes, and most interestingly, in discussing the economic dimension of illicit drugs, only 5 per cent of the articles examined mentioned the word "mafia" (ibid.).

Some of the early critical contributions on drug issues in Italy anticipated debates and controversies that continue today. It was argued by those rejecting traditional accounts that drug use *per se* is not pathological and that intervention should have clear limits (Arnao 1975). Criticism was made, on the one hand, of the media and on the other of prevalent stereotypical attitudes, in their alarmism about illegal drugs alongside misleadingly benign views about legal drugs. The media, it was stressed:

> moralistically reproach the *drug-fiends*, and depict in prud-
> ish tones the sinful atmosphere, the promiscuity, the
> orgiastic deprivation, and the artificial paradise that lurk in
> *drug-parties* (Arnao 1975: 15).

Critical analysis of drug use initially focused on how the phenomenon itself was institutionally and socially perceived – seldom did it explore the individual and collective dynamics of drug abuse or the economic dimension of trafficking and distribution (Blumir 1973). Some authors argued that during the 1950s, drug use in Italy had involved only limited sectors of the "bourgeoisie", so that a limited interest in the problem was largely understandable. Reports from

26

various Court cases of the 1950s were riddled with moral observations regarding the privileged classes who, it was said, abused their social position by indulging in sensual excesses and intemperance: "people who use drugs are pushed by a tremendous anxiety for pleasure and are seduced by the mirage of refined joys, especially with respect to sex" (Insolera & Stortoni 1976: 125).

By contrast, during the 1960s, diffusion of drug use among the younger generations was attributed to the influence of imported youth cultures and styles, and interpreted as a development consistent with the students' struggles and spirit of 1968. Thus, for example, in the prestigious Italian *Dizionario di Sociologia* published in the mid 1970s, the word "drug" appears only twice, each time under the heading "countercultures" (Gallino 1978).

In the late 1970s, with the spread of heroin use, the drug problem was finally perceived as a wider social problem, and this view spawned a relevant and diversified literature. Contributions focusing on the legal aspects of heroin use were followed by ethnographic descriptions of the junkies' underworld (Cancrini et al. 1977, Rusconi & Blumir 1978). Soon afterwards criminological and psychological interpretations added to the jurisprudential knowledge of the subject matter (Di Gennaro 1982). Finally, specific attention was devoted to organized crime which, along with the spread of heroin, made a sensational return to the political and economic stage (Pantaleone 1979).

Some writers noted that, only a few years earlier, what was understood by the term "drug addiction" was addiction to amphetamines or methaqualone: only in the mid 1970s did heroin addiction come to dominate discussion of drug issues (Jervis 1976). In some accounts, the involvement of organized crime in illicit drugs distribution was deemed to be not so much the cause of the spread of heroin, but the consequence of a previously developed drug culture (ibid.). This culture had been fostered by the large and diverse supply of drugs produced by and diverted from the pharmaceutical industry. According to Jervis it is very difficult to draw a neat line between opiates and synthetic drugs, between these and certain analgesics, between certain analgesics and certain hypnotics or sedatives: they may all lead to a habit.

Other authors suggested that heroin use or addiction among Italian users did not follow from the previous or simultaneous use of

27

cannabis, but from a prior history of use of psychotropes like amphetamines (in Italy amphetamines were on sale without prescription until 1972):

> It is apparent that the large spread of the use of licit psychotropes created a custom which can be defined as "toxicophile", and that this has prepared the terrain for the consumption of illicit drugs, particularly of heroin (Bandini & Gatti 1987: 293).

In the mid 1970s, with the drug culture undergoing significant changes, attempts were made to understand its evolution and, *a posteriori*, to pinpoint its different stages. From being an emblem of "affluence" and presumed rebellion, drug abuse rapidly became a symptom of marginalization, especially for young people. This evolution can also be observed both when reading through the data regarding drug use on a national level, and when looking at the findings of locally focused research (Picotti 1979).

However, by the early 1980s, heroin use no longer seemed to be exclusively associated with social marginality, or explainable in terms of social pathology (Labos 1986). Instead, some heroin users were observed to be conducting relatively conformist and orderly lifestyles (Censis 1986). This pattern is still developing. (For data on the epidemiology of opiate and other drug use in Italy during the 1980s see Avico et al. 1990, who estimated that there were 68,000 young male opiate users in 1980 and 92,000 in 1982).

Considering drugs other than heroin, Lewis (1989: 39–41) presents an account of cocaine use and distribution in Rome. Consumption is described as intermittent and recreational, cutting across all social classes, but more erratic in availability and hence forming a much smaller core market, than heroin. Irregularity of supply is possibly related to changes in operations made by the South American groups that dominate the trade. According to Lewis (ibid.) cocaine use is interestingly linked to desirable characteristics of power and sophistication by members of the Rome underworld and hence, along with cannabis, has become their preferred drug. In other cities there are similar indications that cocaine is heavily used by professional criminals (Marozzi & Merzagora 1992).

Only recently has cocaine use raised concern in Italy, although there is widespread belief that the drug *per se* is not dangerous. Research studies in Italy have tended to emphasize that harm is associated with particular social conditions in which cocaine may be used rather than with the drug itself, which is often available on the market at high levels of purity. The literature reports only one death from cocaine overdose between 1986 and 1989 (ibid.). Only 1.5 per cent of drug users known to drug agencies are self-reported cocaine users; but this figure may be a poor indicator of prevalence because of the popularity of the drug among the higher middle classes who can afford private treatment which will conceal them from official records.

Heroin users in Italy rarely resort to cocaine to counter the effects of their main drug. Instead, they are more likely to consume large amounts of alcohol as a depressant drug (Grosso 1992). Availability of cocaine is, therefore, higher than the Italian internal market can absorb. This would suggest that quantities of the drug are being exported out of Italy and into other parts of Europe.

Overall, in Italy, cocaine is widely assumed to be non-addicting, hence discussions of "dependence" and "the drug problem" will focus on heroin. Drug users seem less inclined to use legal drugs, alcohol and pharmaceuticals, than they once were (Arlacchi 1992a) and the imagery and preoccupations of Italian drug culture continue to revolve around heroin and its alleged potency. We shall discuss connections between drug cultures, markets and organized crime below in Chapter 3.

The situation in other European countries

The Netherlands

Between the end of the Second World War and the 1950s, enforcement efforts and seizures indicated availability and use of small amounts of cocaine and morphine, marijuana cigarettes found among crews of US ships, and opium smoking within the Chinese community. In the 1950s, the marijuana trade grew (until 1953 possession and sale were not prohibited by law, De Kort & Korf 1992: 137). As elsewhere, the 1960s were the decade of change, with cannabis and LSD becoming popular and then, in the early 1970s, heroin arriving to become "the problem drug *par excellence* in the Netherlands" (ibid.: 138).

Regarding heroin use in Amsterdam, Korf (1987) suggests that the mid-late 1980s saw a decline or at least stabilization. Samson (1990: 25) notes that 1989 figures gave an estimate of "about 7000 (opioid) addicts in Amsterdam out of a population of 692,000" and reliable estimates for the whole country suggested between 15,000 and 20,000 addicts out of a total population of 14.7 million. Hashish and marijuana use is reported to have been at a fairly stable, low level since the 1970s.

Samson (ibid.: 25–6) suggests that a number of general trends can be identified in describing the patterns of drug use in the Netherlands:

> The extent of the overall problem appears to be stabilising and is even decreasing in some cities; over the years drug abuse seems to have increased among groups in a relatively disadvantaged social and economic position, particularly among ethnic minorities; the use of cocaine is increasing, though not alarmingly so; heroin users tend not to restrict their use to heroin but combine it with other substances, including psychotropic substances and alcohol; the average age of users is rising and today lies between 25 and 35; people are older when they take drugs for the first time.

The heroin available in the Netherlands mainly originates in Iran and Afghanistan, with some coming from the Golden Triangle region. Samson (1990: 42) suggests that domestic drug manufacture includes amphetamine production aimed at sales in the nearby Scandinavian market, domestic demand apparently being "negligible".

Since the 1980s, the question of whether Europe can expect a deluge of cocaine has prompted much concern and study. Some research indicates that cocaine has become more widely available in the Dutch drug scene (Kaplan et al. 1985), though by how much is uncertain and prevalence indicators have been criticized as unreliable (Korf 1987). Whatever the actual prevalence, most researchers argue that cocaine use does not (so far) seem to have given rise to major problems. Cohen's (1989) study of cocaine use in Amsterdam suggests that "support for the hypothesis that the pharmacological characteristics of cocaine make problematic [high] use patterns inevitable was not found. On the contrary, there are no indications that our group of experienced cocaine users lost control and developed into compulsive high level users." On the other hand, a more recent study conducted in Rotterdam (Bieleman & Kaplan 1992; part of an ongoing comparative project also involving researchers in Barcelona and Turin), offers less sanguine conclusions. With a more complex sample (110 respondents, who also provided information about 1051 other users), representing eight different categories of cocaine lifestyles, this research found that "more than half (55%) of the respondents have had problems connected with the use of cocaine" (ibid.: 187). For some users, problems may follow from polydrug use, mixing heroin and cocaine use, and/or being unfamiliar with the rules and rituals that should help avoid problems related to cocaine use. Another study of Rotterdam drug users conducted by Grund (Bockma 1992: 193) "shows that the approximately 3000 users who make up the drugs scene are able to control their heroin use to a certain extent. But the same does not apply to cocaine and that is where most of the problems occur. Many completely lose control of their habit." Significantly, Grund reports that users in his study did not snort but either smoked or injected cocaine, methods of use more like the problematic "crack smoker" style of the USA than the usual "sniffer" described in other Dutch studies.

Drug policy and harm minimization in the Netherlands
The Netherlands has adopted a pragmatic harm minimization approach, most explicitly in recent years though its roots go back to policy foundations laid in the 1970s (and arguably to a "cultural revolution" during the 1960s (Van Vliet 1990)). There is, however, some dispute over how Dutch policy should be characterized. Conservative critics, of course, view it as irresponsibly liberal, while advocates extol its practical virtues (Buning 1992, IJDP 1992a, Engelsman 1989, Baanders 1989), but there are also interpreters of such policy who strongly support its principles but are suspicious of inconsistencies in the motives of some and critical of the way "pragmatism" may turn to "conservatism" (Mol & Trautmann 1991).

The principal enforcement and prevention legislation is the Opium Act 1919. This was amended in 1976 to introduce the basis for the Netherlands' significant (and well known but frequently misunderstood) attempt to differentiate between drug markets. Drugs which present an "unacceptable risk" to society, such as opium, heroin, cocaine, amphetamines etc. are still prohibited and classified under Schedule 1 of the Opium Act, but marijuana and hashish are placed under Schedule 2. Schedule 1 drugs remain heavily penalized, Schedule 2 only moderately so. Part of the rationale for this measure is of particular interest to the theme of this book because it takes a hypothesis about the possibility of separating drug markets as its starting point and builds significant (and apparently successful) legislation upon this. This idea is that cannabis use presents considerably less risk to the individual and society than involvement with other drugs and hence "the dissociation between cannabis use and opiate or amphetamine use should be encouraged by the separation of the illicit markets for these substances. Different penal measures for the unlawful supply of cannabis and 'hard' drugs could contribute to that end" (Samson 1990: 38). It does not appear that tolerance of small-scale cannabis use and open sale in the "coffee shops" has led to any escalation of marijuana use, indeed some reports suggest a decline (Korf 1990, VanVleit 1990, Jansen 1991) – a finding which confounds the criticisms of many overseas commentators.

In 1975 a Government White Paper laid out a policy principle that remains unchanged: drug misuse policy should aim to "contribute to the prevention of and to deal with the risks that the use of mind-altering drugs present to individuals themselves, their immediate environment, and society as a whole." (Samson 1990: 26). Interestingly, Samson argues that formation of such policy has not been the uniquely Dutch product of a culture of tolerance as sometimes portrayed, as if such thinking and arguments have been unrehearsed elsewhere; (see e.g. USA: the Shafer Commission 1972 and 1973; Canada: Report into the Non-Medical Use of Drugs 1973; UK: Wootton Report 1968; WHO: 20th Report of the WHO Expert Committee on Drug Dependency 1974).

It is possible that the well known "Junkiebonden" fraternity of drug users, which has lobbied on behalf of the interests of users in the Netherlands in ways unseen in other countries and with a high profile and high degree of success, reflects a certain particularity about Netherlands culture. This forum has also contributed to the adoption of benign harm minimization policies and practices, notably and very importantly in recent years, in response to AIDS/HIV. Dutch "Junkie Unions" were involved in the first needle exchanges in the country in the early 1980s and have helped pass on public health messages and practices (Kaplan et al. 1986). As with recent policy statements from the ACMD (1988; 1989) in Britain, Dutch policy is clear that "the spread of HIV infection is a greater danger to individual and public health than drug misuse" (Samson 1990: 30), and policy and practice may be having some positive impact (van Haastrecht et al. 1991).

Denmark

As Jepsen (1989: 107) observes, "Danish and Dutch drug policies seem to have much in common, as have criminal and social policies in the two countries in general". A liberal set of attitudes and reluctance to try to "solve social problems through the penal system" underpins Denmark's response to drug problems. This is not without its problems in terms of the discomfort it causes its other European neighbours, "resulting in repeated attacks . . . for being too liberal, thereby creating a risk for Holland and Denmark to become havens for drug traffickers as well as for drug users, creating further risk that traffick and habits may spread to surrounding countries"(ibid.). Denmark's closest neighbours, Norway and Sweden have particularly punitive drug policies and are regularly critical of the Danish approach.

In reality, the Danish drug problem is quite modest and contained. Cannabis is the dominant drug, but morphine, heroin and other opiates are commonly used. LSD seems to have declined in use and while cocaine is available it has not achieved widespread popularity, probably due to its high cost in Denmark. In the late 1980s, amphetamine "entered the Danish drug scene in rather large quantities, most of it imported, other parts derived from legal sources, and in a few instances some of it produced at clandestine domestic laboratories. It has become a very popular drug among young persons, belonging or aspiring to 'the jet set'. It has recently, however, spread also among school children, being preferred to beer or other types of alcohol, due to its euphoriant qualities and its relatively low price ('the poor man's cocaine')" (ibid.: 125).

The most famous area in Denmark associated with drug use and dealing is the so-called "Free city of Christiana" in Copenhagen. Here heroin and other "hard" drugs are easy to obtain while cannabis is sold openly on the streets and squares. But there is evidence that drug use is more widespread in Danish society than in the past. An uncertain estimate of between 5000 and 10,000 "hard core" addicts seems to underpin policy: "the common view is that the rise in this number was halted sometime in the early 70s, as evidenced by the constantly increasing average age of addicts in contact with treatment institutions. In recent years, however, a new wave of younger users may be on the way . . ." (ibid.: 127). The number of drug offenders in prison has seen a constant rise since the 1970s (ibid.: 132), the number of narcotic related deaths increased dramatically between 1968–87 (with peaks around 1980 and 1984), seizures of both heroin and cocaine have been erratic but show overall upward trends between 1978 and 1987 (ibid.: 138), and the price of drugs in the 1980s either remained fairly stable or in some cases (e.g. amphetamine) actually declined (ibid.: 139). The persistence and growth of a drug problem in Denmark may provide support for policy makers who urge a more repressive stance but at the same time, Jepsen notes that there is "a mounting scepticism regarding the possibility of 'eradicating' the drug problem in Denmark through repressive measures" (ibid.: 108). Instead the concept of "control damage" has been introduced, favouring growing use of methadone in treatment, and encouraging a climate of debate in which some form of legalization of cannabis has been discussed – although as Jepsen (ibid.: 128) observes, even in liberal Denmark, any concrete proposals along these lines "will meet with heavy opposition."

Sweden

Sweden differs from other western European countries in that the pattern of drug use which dominates drug policy is not heroin use but the intravenous injection of amphetamine. Hartnoll et al. (1989: 10) note that in

Stockholm, widespread injection of amphetamines since the middle of the 1960s, complemented cannabis use in other groups. The problem culminated at the beginning of the 1970s. Heroin was introduced in the mid-1970s, but was concentrated at Stockholm (and at Malmo, close to Copenhagen). In 1984, the number of injectors in Stockholm was estimated at 3000–4000. Heroin use has never exceeded one third of this population, and in the period 1985–1986, the drug situation seemed to stabilize at a lower level. (see also Jenner 1986: 6–7).

In 1986 Lundborg & Wikman (1986: iv–6) noted a figure of "slightly over 1000 persons" who were heroin abusers. These commentators, from the Swedish Ministry of Health and Social Affairs, observed that "heavy abuse [of drugs generally] outside of the cities is marked by mixed abuse. These abusers use amphetamine, cannabis, prescription drugs, and above all, alcohol" (ibid.).

Unusually, all this makes heroin users a minority. Hartnoll (1986: 68) notes that "although there was a temporary increase in heroin use at Malmo during the late 1970s, there has been no substantial and continued availability or use of heroin" in the country, although Hartnoll et al. (1989: 10) note that in 1987, indicators pointed to a sudden rise in heroin use. While this rise did not amount to the "epidemic" experienced by some other western European countries in the mid 1980s, this may not be cause for a sanguine response to heroin problems in Sweden. In 1986, Lundborg & Wikman (1986: iv–32) observed that Stockholm was "in the middle of an AIDS epidemic among heroin abusers, with approximately 50%" carrying the AIDS virus.

At the end of the 1980s, the injecting population seems to have been "about the same size and found in the same segments of the population as a decade earlier . . . primarily among marginalized groups, such as ex-convicts, institutionalized youth and prostitutes: a subculture that was already heavily criminalized." (Hartnoll et al. 1989: 10–11). So far cocaine does not seem to have made much impact in Sweden or elsewhere in Scandinavia, although during the mid 1980s, concern was aroused in much the same way as elsewhere in Europe. Limited cocaine use seems confined to certain fashionable and other socially well-established groups (Jenner

1986: 13, Lundborg & Wikman 1986: iv–26).

The object of policy in Sweden is a drug-free society: there is no distinction made between soft and hard drugs, criminal law is invoked punitively, prevention, treatment and rehabilitation are emphasized, and compulsory care can be imposed (Lundborg & Wikman 1986: *passim*, Gould 1989). According to Gould (1989: 731), Sweden's "strong temperance tradition has led to an obsession with substance misuse generally, which, in the face of economic difficulties and the fear of AIDS, has resulted in the Swedish version of the new moralism, precipitating harsh, controlling and possibly counterproductive measures." All of this is, as commentators have noted, quite remarkable for at least two reasons: first, increasing repressive policies and further divorcing them from the general trends of other domestic policies is odd given that Sweden's drug problem is limited, and that there are indications that it may be decreasing; secondly, escalating enthusiasm for "the war on drugs" goes against the grain of a tradition of independence in Swedish foreign policy that once stood for reason and for solidarity with developing countries (Lindgren 1992: 104). (Further discussion of drug policy and law in Sweden can be found in Solarz 1989; an interesting comparison of the "restrictive" tendency in Sweden (a case study of Orebro) and a "liberal" one in Britain (a case study of Leicestershire) is found in Gould 1990: 229–50.)

France

It is striking to note that in 1924 Paris had more habitual drug users known to the police than it does today: about 80,000 people were regular users of drugs, mainly cocaine and morphine (de Celis 1992). More recently, figures for the number of opiate users in France *as a whole* have grown dramatically. In 1969 there were 5000–7000 users, in 1971 15,000–20,000 (including an estimate of occasional users). By 1986 heroin was used regularly by some 60,000 individuals, a figure rising further to 100,000 in 1990 (Luckett 1991). Hartnoll et al. (1989: 9) observe that Paris experienced "epidemic growth" in heroin use between 1977 and 1982, with an apparent ageing of users resulting from "the natural aging of existing users and a wider age range of initiation." (A description and discussion of three epidemiological studies carried out in the

Paris region in 1981–82 can be found in Ingold & Olivenstein 1983; see also Facy et al. 1991a,b). Ingold (1985a: 209) records that:

> Up until 1960, very little heroin was consumed in France. True, the "French connection" laboratories were producing very high quality heroin, but almost all of it was exported. The small number of users were to be found in certain limited circles (e.g. those connected with prostitution) and a user who did not "know the ropes" was unlikely to be able to count on regular supplies.
>
> Towards the end of the 1960s, the situation changed completely. A whole new market spread from Marseilles to Paris and other large cities. Heroin was not difficult to acquire and prices were not excessively high. Speaking of that period, one user commented: "In 1968 there were more pushers than junkies and a quarter (of a gramme) only cost 50 francs".

As elsewhere, youth cultures and drugs were linked together in France in the mid 1960s. An association with the student movement, counter-cultures and underground youth magazines (such as *Actuel*; Coluccia 1990) of the period, are all said to have contributed to the spread of drug use. In a 1971 article in *Le Monde* (4 December 1971), certain un-named intellectuals were also blamed for the spread of this "scourge" because they had encouraged the young to despise the values of civilized and democratic French society.

The availability of illegal drugs on the French market is closely associated with the late-colonial nature of French international relations. Throughout the 1950s and 1960s, French drug distributors held a dominant position in international refining and distribution. The "French Connection" and concentration of drug business around Marseilles was the result of – and indeed reflected France's colonial relations. These made the conduct of business between French companies and partners in North Africa and Indochina, a routine matter. Both legal and illegal commerce could flourish and illicit drugs simply followed the same trading channels utilized by legal entrepreneurs (Ruggiero 1986). Such colonial associations may explain the low social status sometimes ascribed to heroin users, particularly involving ethnic minorities from North Africa (Hartnoll et al. 1989: 11).

Intravenous drug users in France are the second largest HIV positive group after homosexuals (Serfaty 1990, see also Facy et al. 1991). Of a sample of 157 street users and 123 persons in treatment, Ingold & Ingold (1989) found 40 per cent were HIV positive. This study aimed to evaluate the effects of liberalization of sale of syringes in 1987–88 and found that while this initiative had an impact on half of the sample, who did not share and bought from pharmacies, the other half continued as before. The need for additional and supplementary educational programmes was therefore noted. According to Ingold (1986: 82) "in general (and particularly after 1975), there [has been] a steady increase in the number of deaths in which heroin was involved; 80% of the deaths related to drug abuse in Paris in 1983 were due to heroin abuse. The number of cases involving volatile solvents and cocaine also increased."

About 60 per cent of the drug users coming to the attention of the criminal justice system have been arrested for cannabis related, not opiate, offences. Seventy per cent of those arrested are aged between 16–25 (Serfaty 1990). The percentage of habitual drug users in French prisons was around 10 per cent in the mid 1980s; if only the larger prisons are considered then this figure had risen to 25 per cent by 1991 (Ingold, et al. 1986, *Rebelles* 1991, Ingold & Ingold 1986).

Recently, a number of French commentators have expressed interest in the relationship between drug use and consumerism. Drug use has been discussed, therefore, against the background of increasing leisure/consumption patterns and the marked individualism prevailing in French society. The strong emphasis on personal achievement and performance has also been attributed an important rôle in creating a "psychotropic culture": a development underlined by the record levels of pharmaceutical purchases in France, the highest in Europe (Ehrenberg 1992). Pharmaceutical products are massively used by all social groups, and commonly regarded as a "chemical crutch" which many rely on to help them through an increasingly competitive and intense urban lifestyle.

Heroin use is also said to be related to this new climate. Users no longer embrace voluntary or involuntary marginalization but express a desire to incorporate their drug use into a normal social life.

Drugs have thus replaced earlier collective and political modes of social expression and socialization as users seek a degree of "normalization" (ibid.).

At the end of the 1980s, Hartnoll et al. (1989: 9) reported that "the most important recent change in drug use (in Paris) was the marked increase in the use of cocaine, as evidenced by the fact that it was being used by all social classes, and some of it was being distributed at the street level". Sellal (1991: 416) remarks that while "cocaine abuse remains limited as compared to heroin addiction . . . the low number of cocaine abusers recorded does not reflect the actual situation, [in part because] some heroin abusers make use of cocaine and this multi-drug use, either regular or occasional, does not appear in the statistics since only the dominating drug is taken into consideration."

Germany

Kreuzer et al. (1991a: 151) note that, even before reunification, Germany could be considered a key "gateway for the narcotic trade due to its central location in Western Europe" and that during the 1980s, drug seizures were reaching "alarming levels". Heroin remains the principal drug of concern but recent attention has also focused on cocaine, especially after 1986 when cocaine seizures outstripped heroin (ibid.: 161). One study, conducted by Kreuzer and colleagues between 1978-80 provides an assessment of drug use and control issues arising in the 1970s, with particular reference to heroin. This study employed life history interviews with 77 arbitrarily chosen "hard drug users", with average ages of 24.1 years for the men and 23 years for the women; only two users were employed at the time of the interview, "for the others, unemployment appeared to be the result and not the cause of their drug career" (ibid.: 152, 153). The drugs used by these respondents mark the "early German hard drug subculture up to the beginning of the 1970s":

> The most important drug for all the respondents was heroin. Almost 90% had experimented with hashish or LSD before advancing to "hard" drugs; the duration and significance of the experimental phase, however, varied from person to person. In 66% heroin had always been the principal

injection drug; 8% started out with *"Berliner Tinke"* (a morphine base dissolved in acetic acid, boiled and injected), 12% with synthetic opiates, and 13% pure opium . . .

In addition to the "soft" drugs . . . the subjects mainly took "speed", "substitute drugs" (barbiturates, Tilidin, and Methaqualone), and, to a lesser degree and in combination with heroin, cocaine. Cocaine, however, is not likely to become as popular as heroin because of its high price and short-lasting effect. (ibid.: 153–4)

The Berlin drug scene developed somewhat earlier than markets in the rest of West Germany, but cities like Hamburg and Frankfurt cannot have been far behind and as Kruezer et al. (ibid.: 155) note, there seem to be few differences between the drug subcultures of Berlin and the rest of (pre-unification) West Germany, or between users who moved from other drugs to heroin and those whose drug use started with heroin.

For Hamburg, Hartnoll et al. (1989: 8) summarize trends in drug use from the early 1970s to the 1980s:

Around 1970, a drug culture comprising users of cannabis and LSD with a middle-class social background emerged at Hamburg. A minority went on to use opiates. In 1974, a heroin market was established. This market has continued, with interruptions, until today. The number of injecting opiate users at Hamburg continued to be stable into the 1980s. Then, in 1987, many indicators pointed to a sharp rise. Survey data suggested a decline from 27 to 14% in the number of persons who had "ever used illegal drugs" (mainly cannabis) at the beginning of the 1980s.

A study of 100 "hard drug addicts" in some kind of detoxification treatment, conducted during the 1980s, provides the following summary of trends in drug use during this decade (Kreuzer et al. 1991a: 158):

. . . it is to be noted that in addition to heroin (the predominant drug) a multitude of other drugs are taken together with or as a substitute for heroin. The use of cocaine has increased sharply; it has developed from a jet-set drug to a street level drug. According to the users questioned here, it is normally not sniffed, but injected intravenously just like heroin. The semi-legal sleeping pills, painkillers and tranquillisers (sometimes prescribed by doctors, but also commonly sold in the drug scene), which are often used in combination with alcohol and heroin (leading to unforeseeable interactions of the individual drugs) are even more significant, especially among women. "Crack" and "designer drugs" have been of no importance so far, at least in the (public) hard drug scene. In certain discotheques it may be different, as some interviews would suggest. "Speed-type" amphetamines, too, play only a subordinate rôle, at least in the Frankfurt area. This corresponds to the findings of the prosecuting authorities.

According to Hedrich (1990: 159) various estimates have been made of the number of intravenous and other drug users in West Germany: "the police have estimated that there are between 50,000 and 60,000 people dependent upon illicit drugs in the FRG, of whom 90% are opiate users . . . Unofficial estimates of the extent of illicit drug use have been far higher."

In discussing the data from their studies, Kreuzer et al. (1991b: 410) offer an interesting consideration of class and age characteristics of German drug users:

At one time it was expected that there would be a shift in the hard-drug scene from a predominance of upper class people to a preponderance of people from lower social classes, but this expectation has not been confirmed. Despite the difficulty in making comparisons with the normal population, there is no proof of any clear tendency towards the upper or lower classes among drug addicts.

The only distinct change that has taken place among drug addicts is that the average [age] has risen to 27.9 years. This is due to the fact that the hard drug scene in the Federal Republic of Germany has been established for 25 years . . . the drug scene is nowadays no longer a homogeneous group in which a feeling of common identity could develop. More than ever before, the only single determining element in the open hard drugs scene seems to be the procurement of drugs. [See Chapters 4 and 5 for comparison with trends in England and Italy].

Since the first known cases of AIDS in Germany in 1980-81, drug related HIV and AIDS have, of course, generated concern and research on drug use and sexual behaviour (Hedrich 1990: 159). One study of drug dependent users in long-term therapeutic facilities, conducted in 1987, found HIV infection rates of 15–20 per cent (ibid.). Kreuzer et al. (1991b: 414–15) report that AIDS has had an impact on injecting – "more attention is now being given to the use of sterile syringes", – but "on the other hand, there seems to have been hardly any influence on the sexual activities of drug addicts, especially those who raise their money through prostitution. There was no indication that prostitution was decreasing or that drug addicts were changing to other ways of raising money to buy drugs."

Hedrich (1990) reviews research carried out in Frankfurt, including work on links between prostitution and drug use behaviours. This study has found that many women finance their drug use through prostitution: within the study group there was a "high level of identified HIV infection", "a lack of social and economic support and . . . poor working conditions . . . Prostitution was perceived in a very negative way". Hedrich concludes that "the top priority for AIDS prevention in relation to the sex industry is to foster and to maintain contacts with drug using prostitutes. Such action should aim to reduce the pressures that encourage unsafe sex and unsafe drug use. Services should not cater only for drug users who are prepared to abstain from drug use. Provision should be flexible and 'user friendly'. This is the only way that this important high-risk group of people will be drawn into counselling and care" (Hedrich 1990: 173).

According to some commentators, Germany's problems with drugs and HIV are not the fault of drug users alone – if at all. Gerlach & Schneider (1992) for example, argue that German policy, research, treatment and practice have generally adhered to an abstinence model – despite critics providing "clear evidence of its inefficiency" (Scheerer & Vogt 1989). Even in the context of HIV/

AIDS, they argue that harm-reduction work is difficult to initiate and Scheerer (1989: 172) is damning of resistance to methadone treatment, especially when it might help minimize risk of exposure to HIV/AIDS, suggesting that such a policy stance almost resembles a form of genocide against drug users. Gerlach & Schneider (1992: 85-6) observe that the diversity of drug research, with different messages and findings, has been ignored in Germany and hence the resistance to methadone maintenance (and other options that would lead to a pluralization of care provision), is uninformed. Hedrich (1990: 160) argues that the long-established "abstinence orientation" of policy "has undergone several changes" with "increasing emphasis upon the provision of support which does not necessarily involve total cessation of drug use". However, such changes do not yet seem to be very far-reaching (law and policy are discussed in some detail by Albrecht 1989).

Nonetheless, in Hamburg, the persistence of a serious heroin injecting problem has encouraged local attitudes towards policy and enforcement that are quite unusual in the German context. As Stourton (1993) reports, after years of dealing with serious drug use, related prostitution and crime – and having no success in reducing the problem,

> the Frankfurt police have come to a conclusion with radical implications: it is the illegal culture that surrounds addiction, rather than the drugs themselves, that destroys the addicts and inflicts such livid social scars on the city. It is a conclusion that is leading Frankfurt's city government, sometimes reluctantly, down the road to legalisation. It has brought in the doctor responsible for addicts in Amsterdam to pilot an experimental programme. It is based on the principle that addiction cannot be cured, and that the primary goal of health policy should be to protect the addicts against disease until they are ready to break their addiction themselves.

Initially this programme involves methadone maintenance, but it is proposed that this be extended to offer the "drug of choice" – in most cases, heroin, on the grounds that this would attract more of the hidden population of users to the clinic. However, this would

43

involve changing the German law to make prescribing heroin legal. Importantly, it seems that opposition to such a proposal will not come from the police: "Approaching the drugs problem with public order in mind, the Frankfurt police have reached the same position as the health authorities. Police Director Philippi says that 15% of the crime in the city is directly associated with drugs. He believes he could clear most of that up almost immediately if they were widely available on prescription – 'Long-term, I see only one chance', he says, 'to approach the addict and to offer him the possibility to get his drugs legally in order to dry out the illegal market.'"

If even the hard-line drugs policy of Germany is beginning to countenance forms of decriminalization or legalization, then this debate could be due for serious re-examination in the 1990s. We shall return to this issue in Chapter 3.

Switzerland

Even in a country with such a generally high level of prosperity, problem drug use has been associated with downward social mobility (WHO 1990). During the 1980s it also saw increased tension between differing law enforcement and public health goals. Relatively speaking, Switzerland and Zurich in particular, have a high incidence of HIV. For some time the city authorities and medical services promoted a tolerance policy that led to the establishment of a de-criminalized zone in a central park of the city – which became famous as "Needle Park". The aim was to create a user-friendly space where medical authorities could pass on clean syringes and harm minimization advice through syringe exchange schemes. To the city police force, however, the park became a magnet for drug users and concentrated problems for the police. They argued that the park attracted

> drug users from all over Switzerland and Europe, with an inevitable rise in crime . . . The contradiction between the strategies of police and city council is evident: "It's politically very hard to carry out a raid when soup is just being dished out" (second-in-command, Zurich police). (*Police Review* 1989: 1656).

The needle park experiment was subsequently brought to an end – probably worsening the prospects for dealing with drug problems in the city, as users now gather in a variety of areas such as railway sidings and other places where it is harder for medical and social work staff to maintain contact (Assignment 1993, Grob 1993, Eisner 1993).

Swiss policy has been quite treatment oriented and only recently begun to develop more diverse models and approaches in response to drug users (e.g. Klingemann 1991; discussion of Swiss law and policy regarding illegal drugs can be found in Schultz 1989).

Austria

Levels of heroin use are low in Austria but opiate preparations are fairly readily available – for example, poppy straw to make a "poppy head soup" is smuggled into the country from Hungary (Watson 1991: 13). Indeed, according to Loimer (1992: 87), "the use and abuse of opiates in Austria are reported on from the earliest findings of poppy seeds in Europe to the morphinism in the nineteenth century and S. Freud's 'cocaine' therapy." The discovery of carbonized poppy seeds in Switzerland indicates that poppy plants were cultivated in the region in Neolithic times but with what purpose is less certain. Commentators writing as far back as 1731 noted the use of white poppy extract to calm crying babies, a tradition that was apparently continued in eastern Austria until the Second World War (ibid.). In the 19th century Austria had considerable experience with drug use – opium itself was regarded as a medicine and misused until the 1830s, morphine was discovered in 1804, used as an analgesic during periods of war and quickly produced many addicts, and finally, eminent physicians such as Freud endorsed use of cocaine (ibid.). However, as elsewhere in Europe, drug problems declined in the early decades of the twentieth century and war and occupation had their own impact.

In the period following the Second World War, long-term prescribing of morphine was the favoured treatment for those who had developed dependence during the conflict, mainly doctors, nurses and war-disabled, and it was not until the 1960s that illicit drug users emerged on any significant scale:

In 1970, the number of drug users was estimated at 10,000; about 500 injected raw opium. Up until today, the number of illegal drug users has been constantly increasing. In 1980, the number of unknown cases must have been 8,000–10,000 heroin addicts. Heroin predominantly comes from the Lebanon and Iran but it is also smuggled from the Netherlands to Austria. Each year, from 1981 to 1988, 4,500–5,500 people were reported to the police for illegal drug abuse or an infraction of the Opium Act . . . : cannabis was abused by two-thirds of the above, opiates and descendents by one-third. Cocaine and the wide variety of other substances remained below 1% in Austria. The number of crimes coming under the Opium Act have also been on the increase. In addition to heroin, "opium tea" is consumed by some Austrian opiate addicts exclusively, or when heroin is difficult to obtain. The opium tea is extracted from dried poppy-heads. Depending on the country of origin they contain a considerable amount of the substances found in raw opium (ibid.: 88).

Methadone maintenance has been legal since 1987, aimed at long-term users who have attempted rehabilitation but not succeeded and at injectors who are HIV positive. In 1989, eastern Austria was reported to have a 30 per cent, and western Austria a 40–50 per cent, rate of HIV infection among drug injectors (ibid.: 89). Harm minimization policies are being encouraged but the prospects for any form of decriminalization are remote (Fehervary 1989: 77–8; this article also provides a useful review of drug law and policy in Austria).

Greece

From around the mid 19th century to the 1970s, drug use in Greece principally involved hashish. Cannabis, cultivated for the production of hashish, was grown in the Peloponnese from about 1875, the techniques being passed on by Greek refugees from Egypt and Cyprus, as well as from other refugees from the East.

Around 1922, hashish consumption in Greece rose considerably for two major reasons: a) the soldiers on the Asia Minor front brought back the habit they had acquired there and, b) the settlement in Greece of immigrants from Asia Minor in very poor economic and social conditions fostered their use of hashish. Until 1960, hashish consumption was confined almost exclusively to the working class . . . (and) until 1970, the ratio of users of other drugs (especially heroin) to hashish smokers was 1:10. (Kokkevi 1986: 1).

During the 1970s, the class and age of users changed, as did the drugs available. Across a range of social classes, the 15–25 year age group became more involved in drug taking – and now for reasons less to do with the traditional associations that hashish use held in working-class cultures, and more to do with imported "western lifestyles" (ibid.: 2). After 1977–8, use of opiates and derivatives, plus cannabis and psychotropes, all increased. Concern and alarm was expressed by the public, church, political organizations and media.

Ingold et al. (1988: 14) draw upon a prevalence study of known cases of drug use and the nationwide general population survey to provide a picture of drug use in Greece during the 1980s (cf. Madianou et al. 1987). The "Prevalence" study was a retrospective review of cases of treated or recorded drug users covering the period 1973–83. Describing this study, Kokkevi (1986: 3) notes that "according to the data collected, the number of registered cases in 1983 is 9689 addicts. Most of them (91%) are male. The number of female addicts increases significantly after 1976. The main age for both sexes presents a significant decrease during the 1973–83 period." Ingold et al. (op. cit.) also summarize data from this study:

the mean age for male drug users was 35.7 and for female drug users 31.2. The study revealed [findings that imply] that a substantial number of drug users have migrated to the Greater Athens area . . . Of the known cases, 61% of males and 50% of females had been involved in illegal activities other than drug related ones. The great majority of them had been arrested once (90%) but only 14% of them had been sentenced to imprisonment. Among males, the most frequently used drug was cannabis (53.3%) followed by heroin and other opiates (27.9%). Among females heroin was at the first place (51.2%) followed by cannabis (30.3%). (ibid.: 14–15).

Kokkevi (1986: 4) also comments that "there is . . . extensive criminal activity, since 90% of the population (in the study) had been arrested and convicted on charges other than drugs. Furthermore an important increase in arrests and hospitalisations has been observed during the ten years."

Overall in Greece, rising figures for numbers of drug users, continued increases in seizures of drugs between the late 1970s and late 1980s, an increase in deaths by overdose in the mid-late 1980s (Ingold et al. 1988: 16) and growing demand for counselling and places in therapeutic communities (Manou 1992), all suggest a worsening drug problem.

Kokkevi (1986: 7–10) observes that it is only relatively recently that Greece has had such a drug problem to respond to. New legislative, prevention and rehabilitative measures have, therefore, been promoted. These include a low key response to non-dependent first offenders scaling up to compulsory or voluntary enrolment in therapeutic programmes for dependent users, and increasing prison penalties for traffickers. Prevention and rehabilitation issues seem to have been particularly strongly emphasized in Greece.

Spain

In Spain, problems relating to illegal use of drugs are also relatively recent, with significant increases only occurring in the 1980s (Alvarez & Del Rio 1991:70). Epidemiological data are limited but general trends can be discerned (ibid.; WHO 1992). The most popular drug in Spain is cannabis but other drugs used include amphetamines, heroin, cocaine and hallucinogenics. In 1989, 47 per cent of seizures were of cannabis, 32 per cent opiates and 12 per cent cocaine; in the same year, 96 per cent of admissions to treatment involved heroin, 2.5 per cent other opiates and 1.7 per cent cocaine. In recent years arrest rates have doubled, seizure of drugs tripled and amounts confiscated increased: "based on these indicators, the consumption of cannabis has decreased and that of opiates, cocaine and other substances has risen" (WHO 1992: 79). According to data from the State Information System for Drug Abuse covering 1987–89,

> the average age of treated drug users increased [from 24,1 to 25,3] which possibly reflects the *ageing of opiate and cocaine users*. The average age of initial consumption was approximately 20 years and remained practically stable. First cocaine use and treatment admission occurs at a higher age than in the case of heroin . . . the male/female ratio remained constant (4:1) [and] survey data indicated that only the consumption of tranquillizers and hypnotics is higher among women than among men (WHO 1992: 79; emphasis in original).

Data for the city of Barcelona (Ingold et al. 1988: 20–21) suggest that during the 1980s the rate of admission to treatment increased, especially at the beginning of the decade; drug related deaths increased significantly between 1970 and 1987, jumping from two to 50 cases; drug seizures, police arrests and cautions and other indicators of rising drug use, have all increased. Between 1983 and 1985 the majority of hospital emergency room cases that were drug related involved heroin use. In the mid to late 1980s, it was noted that a rise in cocaine related episodes had occurred (ibid.: 21). Alvarez & Del Rio (1991) note that data from the areas of Castile and Leon also show significant increases in cocaine use, while Torrens et al. (1991: 29) have specifically examined the rise in use of cocaine by heroin addicts and argue that "multiple data suggest that Spain is suffering a new era of epidemic dimensions with regard to the consumption of cocaine. Direct and indirect indicators, such as confiscations, health problems in emergency rooms and number of patients seeking treatment in drug addiction services, indicate the existence of an increasing population of cocaine consumers." The authors argue that this may be particularly worrying in relation to prevalence of HIV because "dual addiction to intravenous cocaine and heroin may increase the risk of AIDS, both through needle sharing and through the combined immunosuppressive effect of both drugs" (ibid.: 32).

In 1990, 68 per cent (n=3607) of all registered AIDS cases were intravenous drug users or related groups (WHO 1992: 79). Between

1985 and 1990, deaths from adverse reactions to drugs (particularly heroin), almost tripled (from 143 to 455). Treatment capacity has increased significantly in this period and shows a trend towards outpatient/non-residential care, reflecting rising costs, especially in relation to HIV/AIDS cases (ibid.: 80).

Legislation concerning illegal drugs makes a distinction between soft and hard drugs, and drug consumption *per se* is not penalized, but revisions in the law since 1988 have increased various penalties, notably those for trafficking. Detailed discussion of relevant criminal law and social policy in Spain can be found in de la Cuesta (1989) and Diez-Ripolles (1989a).

Portugal

According to Ribeiro (1986) there is some degree of consensus that an increase in drug taking in Portugal "occurred with the opening of its geographical, political and cultural frontiers, after 25 April 1974", and the re-establishment of democracy, the end of colonial wars and the return of expatriates. Unlike France at the end of its colonialism, Portugal experienced all this during a period of economic recession and increasing unemployment (Ribeiro 1986: 1). With the breaking down of the traditional "social defences" of the previous authoritarian regime, politicians, the military and others, sought an alternative state led response to the new drug problems, emphasizing both prevention and repression (ibid.: 1–2).

A confused and divided set of responses were established that seem to have been wholly unprepared for a sudden and dramatic rise in heroin use which, from 1980, "swamped the whole state control and prevention system" (ibid.: 2). Ribeiro observes that most epidemiological and sociological studies conducted have severe limitations. Dias & Polvora (1983) have reported on a study of 5419 adolescent drug users who came to the attention of three regional drug prevention centres, in Lisbon, Oporto and Coimbro, during the period 1978–81. In this sample:

> 65% were in the 15–21 age group or younger; 57% were male and 43% were female. Among 4,338 drug abusers classified by the type of drug used, cannabis was the most frequently abused (33%), followed by opiates (24%), bar-

biturates (13%), amphetamines (11%), hallucinogens (7%), alcohol (5%), cocaine (4%) and others (3%) (Dias & Polvora 1983: 81).

In the mid 1980s, estimates of the number of heroin addicts in the country were considered "unreliable and contradictory", ranging from 10,000 to 65,000, and looking to the future a picture of poor co-ordination and instability was predicted for services and other responses to Portugal's drug problems (Ribeiro 1986: 4–8).

Ireland

Reporting on drug use trends in the Republic of Ireland, between 1968 and 1978, Corrigan (1979) suggested that the country had been fortunate and had experienced relatively little abuse of dangerous drugs, such as heroin. However, at the time of publication and into the 1980s, Ireland, and Dublin in particular, experienced "an alarming increase in drug abuse among young people" (Corrigan 1986: 91). As O'Kelly et al. (1988: 35) report:

. . . prior to 1979 serious drug abuse was little known in Irish society. It was confined to a small group of addicts whose supply of drugs was unorganized and constantly changing. Drugs used consisted mainly of amphetamines and barbiturates and were obtained on prescription or stolen from chemists shops or pharmacies. Organized drug pushing did not exist. However, in the 1970s there was an increase in the non-medical use of synthetic opiates, Diconal (dipipanone) and Palfium (dextramoramide), and following the increased availability of heroin in the United Kingdom and Europe, the drug scene changed dramatically. There was a rapid increase in the use of heroin by injection in Dublin, particularly in Central Dublin.

Between 1979 and 1983, the number of heroin and other opiate addicts seeking treatment increased four to five times, and there were significant increases in reports of Hepatitis B and of drug-related deaths (Corrigan 1986: 91).

Two field-work studies were carried out in different parts of Dublin in the early 1980s to gather data on users and non-users. Dean et al. (1983) examined trends in a part of the northern inner city of Dublin and found approximately 10 per cent of 15–24 year olds had tried heroin. Comparing users with non-users (matched by age and sex), Dean et al. (1984a) found that heroin users smoked more (twice as many cigarettes), but drank less alcohol. However, heroin users had a greater tendency to come from families where one or both parents had a history of alcohol problems. It was also more likely that their parents had separated or there had been a death of a parent at an early age. Heroin users were unlikely to be employed but this must be seen in a context of high unemployment, with 50 per cent of the non-users also unemployed (Dean, et al. 1984a, Corrigan 1986: 94–5). A study in a suburb in the south of Dublin found only 29 users, or 2.2 per cent, of a population of young people numbering 1327. Similar risk factors were identified in this study, including broken marriages/family backgrounds, premature parental death and alcohol misuse in the family (Dean et al. 1984b, Corrigan 1986: 95).

Overall, Hartnoll et al. (1989: 8) summarize the experience of Dublin thus:

> The first wave of drug misuse occurred . . . in the period 1969–70 and involved mainly amphetamines, barbiturates and cannabis. Heroin was introduced late in the 1970s and an approximate fivefold increase was observed between 1979 and 1983. In 1983, the problem peaked and has since stabilized at a lower level. The evidence suggested that Dublin was the main city in Ireland to experience a severe opiate problem . . . one estimate suggested that in 1985 there may have been about 1700 opiate misusers in the city.

O'Kelly et al. (1988) follow on from the earlier studies by Dean et al. and describe "the rise and fall of heroin use in an inner-city area of south Dublin" between 1979 and 1985. They identify similar risk factors but also draw out broader indices of social deprivation as the background to heroin use in this particular locality – "The Ward". We shall refer to this case study further in considering the issue of social deprivation and drug use below. However, there is one further issue that this more recent work raises and that is HIV/AIDS (ibid.: 37).

The issue of policy and health responses to HIV/AIDS is particularly complex in the case of the Irish Republic. In their excellent article on women, drugs and HIV in Ireland, Butler & Woods (1992: 51) have pointed out that the context is one in which "officials" of the Catholic church "have succeeded to a degree that is unparalleled in other Western societies in limiting and dominating public discourse on a wide range of social policy issues, particularly in the area of sexual morality." More specifically, "Irish responses to HIV and AIDS must be considered against the background of the country's long-standing social policy on marriage, sexuality and reproduction, and its more recent policies on drug problems" (ibid.: 52). Restrictive legislation and practice regarding sex education, contraceptive aids and health education broadly, and "unusually narrow and uncompromising" approaches to treatment and rehabilitation, have made it very difficult for HIV workers to initiate harm reduction services (ibid.: 53–4). From the mid to late 1980s, some progress was made in this direction, with the establishment of a few specialist projects, the availability (for some) of methadone maintenance and the employment of counsellors and outreach workers. However, the account offered by Butler & Woods (1992) suggests that services are still limited and attitudes may have changed only grudgingly (where they have changed at all).

Eastern Europe:

Poland

In contrast to parts of the former Soviet Union, it appears that in pre-war Poland, use of narcotic drugs was rare (Watson 1991: 12). Ethyl ether was prepared in various mixture forms and used particularly in southern regions of the country while in Warsaw "users recruited mostly from the artistic and high life milieux" were linked with some use of morphine, heroin and cocaine (Chrusciel 1990: 10). The main category of known users were registered therapeutic users, a category supplemented after the war by the addition of medical professionals who had abused their access to pharmaceutical supplies. Generally, Polish users have had to innovate and have used a variety of substitutes for narcotic type drugs (Kala &

Borkowski 1990: 129). As Crusciel (op. cit.) summarizes "until the 1960s, experimental, non-dependent drug use generally prevailed. Psychotropic drugs and stolen analgesic drugs were used; non-medical dependent drug use was incidental. Some limited use, including occasional dependent drug use, involved artists, painters, sculptors and other creative personnel as well as some medical personnel. Youngsters and young adults were usually not involved."

A degree of liberalization coinciding with the spread of counter culture ideas, was associated with some slow increase in drug use among young people, particularly those in their late teens – but not by patterns of use characteristic of western Europe or the US. Instead, Poland produced a home grown variety of opiate and related problems.

As Watson (1991: 12) observes, the late 1960s saw the emergence of some demand for recreational drugs – but generating supply was difficult under "economic conditions which sealed the country off from the international drugs market more effectively than any supply control policy could possibly do . . . The non-convertibility of Polish currency acted as a barrier to imports of all kinds, including drugs." The events that changed the Polish drug scene are reputed to be the activities of a chemistry student in Gdansk in 1976, who developed and popularized a simple method of extracting active opiate substances from poppy straw – a home brewing of "makiwara" for oral use and "Kompot" for intravenous use. The procedure spread widely in Poland and subsequently in other countries in eastern Europe (Watson 1991: 12, Crusciel 1990: 10–11). Poppy straw is a waste product of opium poppy grown for seed on many plantations: in the 1970s–1980s "approximately 700,000 farmers cultivated these plantations for the poppy grain" harvested for its nutritional value (Crusciel 1990: 11). Plantations were not subject to any control, farmers were apparently unaware or preferred to appear unaware of potential harm following from allowing access to their crops and waste. It was considered a lucrative, legitimate perk to accept a fee from young people who came in large numbers in the season to collect opium poppy milk (Chrusciel 1990: 11). As drug abuse was a symptom of decadent and corrupt capitalist society and communist society did not face such problems, media and health discussions made no reference to the issue. Psychiatric services, on the other hand, were "acutely aware of the problem" (Chrusciel 1990: 11), although epidemiological data was at first only incompletely collected.

The illegal marketing of opium poppy extract preparations – referred to as "Polish heroin" (although early versions probably contained codeine and morphine, and only later heroin) contributed to the spread of drug abuse in Poland in the 1980s. The late 1970s had seen availability meeting domestic demand but did not appear to produce any marked rise in levels of use, or escalation of demand. Market stability seemed to prevail. However, in the turbulent years of the rise of Solidarity, opiate use gained in popularity. In 1980-81 members of the manual working class were confronting the state, they were also, apparently, turning to home grown opiates (Watson 1989; WHO 1990). This period also saw the simultaneous development of therapeutic community and counselling services, partly organized by a number of students involved in the Solidarity movement who organized MONAR, the Youth Movement to Fight Drug Abuse (Chrusciel 1990: 17).

In a market which until recently resisted commercialization, equilibrium seems to have returned remarkably quickly following this increase in use and Watson (1989) has reported that further increases in the 1980s were negligible despite problems commonly associated with rising drug use – "continuing and dramatic rises in levels of poverty, unemployment, homelessness and crime" (Watson 1991: 13)

Epidemiological and enforcement data also cover increases in use of other drugs in Poland since the 1970s, including anxiolytics, sedatives, hypnotics and illicitly manufactured amphetamines. Tobolska-Rydz (1986) notes that some of the "home-made laboratories" involved in processing poppy straw, also produced methamphetamine hydrochloride and LSD. Cannabis, at one time apparently unpopular and rarely reported, was well established by 1989. As in many parts of western Europe, a pattern of polydrug use now seems to have emerged in Poland – the opiate "compotte" containing morphine, acetylmorphine and heroin remaining a main drug, but now used alongside or interchangeably with various psychotropic drugs, principally benzodiazepines and barbiturates, depending on availability within the illegal market (Chrusciel 1990: 12). Available data suggests that the "typical" Polish drug user is male, of working-class, town origin, with poor educational background, below 30 years and single. At the beginning of the decade there may have been between 80,000 to 200,000 regular and irregular drug users in Poland (ibid.: 13).

Policy in Poland

The principal legislation in force is the Prevention of Drug Abuse Act (30 January 1985). This covers opiates, cannabis and psychotropics and is underpinned by a primary objective, as the title suggests, of preventing drug use/problems (Chrusciel 1990:13). Chapter 5 of the Act covers penal sanctions but use and possession of drugs are not, in themselves, penalized. Drugs are only authorized for certain persons and certain circumstances (e.g. therapeutic purposes; involvement in research). Poland acceded to the Hague Convention in 1922 and to other international agreements up to and including the 1961 and 1971 Conventions (ibid.: 15).

Hungary

According to Levai (1991), developments concerning drugs and drug abuse in Hungary reflect those occurring in other countries of central and eastern Europe, under and after Communism:

> Over the last twenty five years, several tens of thousands of the 10.5 million people living in Hungary have abused drugs in some way. Some represent a broader social movement and some are isolated individual users. Those in the former category are mainly younger people who have got involved in the recent wave of drug abuse; some are regular abusers but many, like in the west, use but do not get dependent on drugs. Young abusers achieve the desired narcotic state by inhaling organic solvents (around fifty deaths from solvent abuse have been proven) and by abusing medicines. With greater western influence however, the knowledge and consumption of a broader range of drugs is taking place. Indeed drugs abuse can increasingly be seen, as in the west, as a "chemical loophole to an antisocial way of life and is at the same time the symbol of dissatisfaction with traditional values." The use of drugs is one of the ways young people seek to embrace the new and abandon the old ideology.

The other group of abusers are adults. They tend to be isolated and not part of a broader social movement like their younger counterparts: many of them are addicts. Their abuse of medicines often leaves them completely isolated but, because of their marginal position, they do not have significant impact on the rest of society.

Hungary is opening up to the drug trade but at the beginning of the 1990s, it is not yet a "target" for such trade, nor is there yet a drug manufacturing network in operation within the country – however, the convertibility of the forint (the national currency) and strengthening of the economy may change things (Lipiay 1992: 71). Illegal use of drugs in the country has been known since the 1960s but the problem was unacknowledged, partly for political reasons but also, according to Lipiay (ibid.: 72) , because there was a belief that drawing attention to the problem might encourage further use. Since the 1980s, there has been some liberalization in treatment methods but the criminality of drug use is also emphasized.

Russia

As Inciardi (1987: 329) reminds us, for well over a generation it was "the position of Soviet officials that opiate addiction and the abuse of other drugs are Western phenomena, natural outgrowths of unemployment and the unequal distribution of wealth that characterize capitalist societies. In a 1971 report to the United Nations (cited by Bruun et al. 1975), for example, a representative from the Soviet Union emphasized that 'as in previous years, drug addiction is not a public health problem . . . this is due primarily to the general social and economic conditions prevailing in the Soviet Union and to the special measures generally taken by the Soviet Government.'" While this may seem a remarkable accomplishment, Inciardi observes that there were good grounds for assuming that there was some truth in these claims: high rates of alcoholism were known but no mention was made by commentators of drug problems, and in a society where totalitarian social control was assumed to be so tight, then the possibilities for widespread trafficking or drug subcultures to flourish looked slim.

With the opening up of Soviet society and the *perestroika* process initiated by Gorbachev, reports and acknowledgements of a sizeable drug problem suddenly emerged. However, it is unclear quite how long the history of this problem may be. On the one hand some observers suggest that widespread drug abuse is relatively new in Russia, and a consequence of two factors. First, the exposure and addiction of Soviet troops to heroin and other drugs while stationed in Afghanistan; secondly, the search for alternative intoxicants when Mr Gorbachev initiated a "war on alcoholism". On the other hand, there has been widespread cultivation of the poppy for generations. As in Poland and Austria, the seeds have been used for various culinary purposes but it would be strange to find that they have not also been used to make opiate drugs (Inciardi 1987: 330). Levai (1991) notes that "according to one estimate by a Soviet state official, more than 50% of the authorized (hemp and poppy) crop is left in the fields after harvest. This 'forgotten' crop is the main source both for abusers and for traffickers." Inciardi (1987: 330) points to the

critical importance, [of] the Soviet Unions' proximity to what has become known as the "Golden Crescent", an arc of land stretching across South-west Asia through sections of Pakistan, Iran and Afghanistan. The Golden Crescent is the primary cultivation area for opium poppies, and it contains a number of the world's most efficient heroin refining and trafficking centres. The Soviet Union borders on much of the Golden Crescent territory, and history has documented time and again that wherever illegal drugs are produced and trafficked they are invariably used by many of those living in the immediate and surrounding areas. (ibid.).

Even more recently, further dramatic changes in the former Soviet Union and Eastern Bloc have broken up the old Soviet empire, removed centralized controls, and brought numerous social, economic and political problems. The breakdown of pervasive social controls, economic instability and unemployment, rising rates of crime, and social malaise generally, have proved fertile ground for social problems, including the growth of forms of "organized crime" and drug use and trafficking (see for example Bohlen 1993, Clark 1993). As Lee (1992: 178)) observes:

Although the [former] Soviet Union is not yet in the midst of a drug epidemic, clear indications suggest that the market for morphine, heroin, hashish, and other illicit substances is expanding in the USSR. The increasing number of Soviet economic and financial ties with the West undoubtedly will accentuate this trend. . . . Moreover, such contacts will surely accelerate the flow of Western narc-expertise – especially in the manufacture and supply of illicit drugs – to Soviet criminal networks. Consequently, the USSR could well assume the rôle of a major player in the international narcotics traffic in the 1990s, as both a consuming and an exporting nation.

One estimate of the number "who have tried drugs or used them" totals "around 1.5 million", extrapolating from a figure of 130,000 registered users and addicts known in 1989. Lee (1992: 178–80) draws upon reports produced from the late 1980s to 1990 to provide a profile of "the average Soviet drug user": "male, less than 30 years of age, a blue-collar worker (in industry, construction, or transport), and fairly well educated".

Principal drugs used during the late 1980s and into the early 1990s are hashish-marijuana (covering different strengths and varieties), Koknar (ground-up poppy straw), and opium. Over such a vast territory there will naturally be regional variations, thus for example, in 1984–5, morphine was reported to be the second most widely used drug in the Georgia area (Lee 1992: 182, see also Inciardi 1987). Heroin is relatively uncommon, with opium being far more widely available, and – as in Poland – home brewed opiate-type preparations, such as koknar and khimka, being popular (Lee 1992: 182).

Russia and other parts of eastern Europe are reported to be particularly at risk of seeing the practice of injecting drugs spread among drug users. An increase in the sharing of needles, with the consequent health hazards this brings, has been predicted (Stimson 1992; *International Journal on Drug Policy* 1992b: 117). A rather more bizarre form of health hazard may be posed to users if reports of opium and marijuana cultivation within a 30 kilometre radius of the Chernobyl nuclear accident are true. A Moscow based group, the International Association to Combat Drug Trafficking and

Abuse, reports that "large quantities of poppies have been seized by police in the area", with plant heads that are "abnormally large". The new drug markets of eastern Europe are presumed to be the destination for the radioactive drugs (*International Journal on Drug Policy* 1992b: X; Boseley 1993; ch. 3 below).

Treatment approaches have been conservative and the introduction of new methods and perspectives is difficult when new resources are unavailable and the specialists of the old order are still in influential positions. Fleming et al. (1992: 28) have reported on the state of drug services in Russia at the beginning of the 1990s:

> The treatment of substance misuse is based upon the state system of narcological clinics which have been set up over the past ten years as narcology has developed as a separate discipline. Narcology embraces all forms of substance abuse. Treatment is aimed mainly at alcoholism, with smoking and drug addiction taking second place. A substance is deemed to be a narcotic if it is on the list of officially proscribed drugs. The Soviets subscribe to the disease model of addiction.

Conventional treatment is, therefore, medically-oriented and hospital based, dominated by psychiatry and psychology. However, there are also alternative therapeutic approaches in use, including acupuncture (which is highly regarded in the Russian medical system), and the establishment of Alcoholics Anonymous groups has brought the "Twelve Steps" model into use. There are few community oriented or based services for drug users except insofar as the police have been expected to perform some unexpected rôles. As Fleming et al. (1992: 29) observe: "the role of the police is extremely complex and somewhat contradictory; on the one hand it is the agency which implements the punitive approach to drug users (through the application of the penal law), on the other hand it has a more humane response to drug use than is sometimes found in the medical profession itself." The issues of AIDS/HIV, syringe exchange and harm minimization do not yet seem to have a high priority place on the new Russian agenda, but it is accepted that official estimates of HIV rates are under-estimates and policy and practice will, no doubt, turn to these issues in time.

Social deprivation and drug use in Europe

In the west, and now increasingly in eastern Europe, commentators have often associated increases in drug use with broader social problems, typically social deprivation, high unemployment, economic dislocation and social marginalization. However, despite common reference to such explanations, the relevant literature does not seem as large as one might expect. Of course, this relationship is by no means straightforward and indeed some would argue that any sort of relationship remains unproven. Furthermore, it may be that the very relevance of the idea of "unemployment" is questionable with regard to the involvement of some – or many – in the drug economy. If people are not without "jobs", but are actually working in the drugs economy and earning considerably more than they might in no-future, low-grade labouring or service jobs, then how appropriate are social policies based on assumptions about the intrinsic desirability of legal work over illegal work? If "market forces" have triumphed, why is it surprising to find people pursuing activities in a market that offers high returns?: "'Why should I work in McDonalds for $4.75 an hour when I can earn two, three thousand dollars dealing drugs?' Tito, a San Francisco gang leader, is the living embodiment of a market principle . . ." (Stourton 1993: 2)

Most studies in this area have sought to examine the evidence for some kind of causal or correlated relationship between deprivation and drug use/dealing and it is probably the latter argument that has been most convincing, whether elucidated by qualitative (Pearson 1987a,b) or quantitative research (Peck & Plant 1986). But such studies have generally focused on the experience of particular areas within individual nations (eg. Unell 1987, Haw 1985, Pearson et al. 1987) and there seems to have been very little work of a comparative nature.

One exception to this is Ingold et al. (1988) who examined the available research literature on polydrug use and "multiple deprivation" in Athens, Barcelona and London. Two of the key questions for this review were: "1) does poverty stimulate the development of drug use in a given community and 2) does poverty influence the outcome of therapeutic and preventive initiatives in a given community?" (ibid.: 2). The term "polydrug" use was chosen to cover a range of drugs including alcohol, and the definition of "multiple deprivation" employed drew on the work of Townsend, (1987). Multiple deprivation denotes more than simple poverty:

> people can be said to be deprived if they lack the material standards of housing, diet, clothing, household facilities, working and environmental facilities . . . which are ordinarily available in the society in which they live. They may also be said to be deprived if they do not have access to forms of employment, education, recreation, and family and social relationships which are commonly accepted. The former may be termed "material deprivation" and the latter "social deprivation" (ibid.).

The case of Dublin in Ireland is one location cited in the study as an example where developments clearly raised the question of links between "(i) availability of drugs, (ii) social distress (and) (iii) drug epidemics." The report notes that between 1979 and 1985 Dublin experienced "a major heroin epidemic" located primarily in the centre of the city and, more precisely, an area known as The Ward. Between 1930 and 1971 this area of the city had lost about 50 per cent of its population, leaving a large proportion of elderly people with low incomes. Housing conditions were poor, with 30 per cent of the population living in overcrowded conditions. Eighty seven per cent of the heroin users had started use between 1977 and 1981:

> they were young (57% under 25), single (76%), unemployed (87%), and usually living with parents or a partner (78%). Many of the women had children and had been using heroin during pregnancy. Educational achievement was usually very low. A large majority of subjects (77%) had served prison sentences, the average length of time spent in jail being 3.4 years. Heavy alcohol use among them and their parents was frequent. Heroin use was highest in 1981 when 9.3% of the population aged 15–24 in the area were using heroin. (ibid.: 8–9; see O'Kelly et al. 1988).

The evidence for an association between local conditions of multiple deprivation and rising heroin use is obviously not conclusive but there would seem to be grounds to assert that there is some strong relationship here. What strengthens this suggestion is that the decline in heroin use, first beginning around 1982, coincided with attempts to improve local social conditions. Decreased use may have been partly related to a possible decline in drug availability but also seems to have been "clearly associated" with "intensive community efforts in the direction of better housing, recreational programmes for youth, training courses for community leaders and a number of local activities" (ibid.: 9).

On the basis of an examination of research materials concerning Athens, Barcelona and London, Ingold et al. (ibid.: 27–8) argue that:

> Multiple deprivation and different forms of drug use are in close relationship even if this relationship is not totally understood. We believe however that these populations which are deprived/marginalized/addicted/involved in more or less criminal activities may be considered otherwise than from an exclusively economic point of view. It implies for the subjects a way of life where the day to day survival becomes part of the picture: being obliged to look for drugs or basic resources every day is not without effects on other problems or aspects of life . . .
>
> Along the same lines . . . the drug addict has to deal with difficulties which are related to an economic dependence (Ingold 1985b), that is to say the structure of drug distribution itself. To be part of the drug distribution network helps the drug user to maintain his habit but it also leads him into an involvement from which there is little hope of escape. From this point of view, the drug addict is more or less inevitably involved in a process of dependence and deprivation which are linked together (ibid.).

The authors concluded that

> in each city, we can say that (a relationship between alcohol/drug use and multiple deprivation) can be established. *But* many questions still remain unanswered and we cannot say there is a straightforward causal link between the two

phenomena. For instance, when we find that drug using individuals are more likely to live in deprived areas, this does
not automatically imply that they are themselves deprived
or with a background of multiple deprivation; an unknown
proportion of them may have moved to a deprived area for
different reasons, including the access to drug supply and
drug markets (ibid.: 31).

This possibility has also been suggested by Forsyth et al. (1992)
in their examination of spatial variations in patterns of drug use in
Glasgow and associations with deprivation, crime and so on. They
note that a number of studies have

> reported finding intra-urban differences in numbers of
> known drug users, generally identifying those neighbour-
> hoods with the greatest number of known drug users as be-
> ing located within some of the most socioeconomically
> deprived areas of a city . . . Drug use, crime and measures
> of urban deprivation have all been found to exist at high
> levels in the same areas . . . In fact, it has been stated that
> all forms of social pathology (including drugs and crime)
> correlate, and therefore, occur in the same neighbour-
> hoods. (ibid. 292).

However, the fact that

> drugs are often linked with deprivation and crime, [is an]
> association [that] may in part derive from where drugs are
> sold, rather than who takes them. Just as American drink-
> ers in the Prohibition era tended to consort with gangsters
> and frequent disreputable speakeasies, so the drug users of
> today are most visible in the deprived areas where they go
> to score. Counting drug users present in deprived areas is
> liable to exaggerate their prevalence, because many live
> elsewhere. . . . When prevalence is exaggerated it then be-
> comes increasingly tempting mistakenly to blame deprived
> areas' numerous problems on drug use and drug users.
> (ibid.: 306)

Thus, Forsyth et al. indicate that there are two directions in which a causal relationship could flow: first, experiencing multiple deprivation in a poorly resourced environment could encourage drug use; secondly, the initiation and then serious spread of drug use in an area could lead to or exacerbate localized socioeconomic problems. Pearson (1987b) neatly describes how, in practice, the two processes are likely to interact (see also Mirza et al. 1991).

Debates about deprivation and deprived classes (now fashionably termed "the underclass") and about drug use as strongly correlated with poverty and marginalization, are important not just in terms of the epidemiology of drug use and health and social work responses. For, depending on the political climate, such debates and arguments can excite or justify responses to drug users which are either benign or quite the opposite. At present, and following much of the American lead in use of the term, western European responses to an underclass are not generous. EC social legislation may seek to extend rights and welfare but the poor, the guestworkers, the non-citizens and the undesirables of society still face what Dahrendorf (1987) calls "The erosion of citizenship" and its entitlements. The underclass have been represented, on the one hand, as "Losing Out" (Field 1989) partly through circumstances beyond their control and, on the other hand, as "idle, thieving bastards" (Bagguley & Mann 1992). Certainly, in Britain, the drug users at the bottom of the social pile join others who are merely estimates in the official statistics on the homeless, the lost and the growing number of itinerant travellers: in Britain, as in other parts of western and now eastern Europe, there are signs of widening gaps between social classes (Townsend 1990, Ingold et al. 1988: 22 and *passim*). Liberal social policy is concerned to ensure that the social welfare net can still catch and assist those who are losing out; conservative policies favour self-help and a dose of old-fashioned "victim blaming". To usefully intervene in the drugs/deprivation relationship, one of these approaches may be helpful – the other will not!

3

Trafficking, markets, crime
and control issues in Europe

In the 19th century, international trafficking in opium and cocaine was a legitimate, state sponsored enterprise for the British and the Dutch, (Berridge & Edwards 1981, De Kort & Korf 1992, Chambliss 1977). This fascinating history cannot be recounted here but it is important to be aware of the *ironies* of history – that states, now signatory to international control conventions, were once traffickers themselves, deriving considerable profit from the drug trade and even employing the forces of warfare to ensure its continuation (Inglis 1976).

The usual way of looking at today's patterns of trafficking assumes that drug producing countries are flooding western societies with dangerous drugs. However, we ought to emphasize that the exporting of dangerous practices has continued to take place in the opposite direction. The forms of processed drugs popular in the west, and western styles, fashions and cultures of use, have all been exported to the producer countries. These countries generally have a long history of recreational, medical or religious drug use, and only recently have they developed patterns of problematic use. The emergence of such patterns is due, in large part, to the export of western drug processing and distribution techniques, which have distorted traditional relationships with indigenous plant drugs. Peasants, hill farmers, Indian tribes and others may maintain such traditions (White 1989) but the urban experience is changing. Just a few decades ago, drugs in these producer countries had a low exchange value and a high use value. Increased involvement in the whole process of transformation, from raw material to refined drug, has meant a dramatic increase in the local availability of processed drugs and the spread of use. Drug entrepreneurs and corrupt officials in these countries now know very well that it is the exchange value of drugs which is all, whereas their use value is nothing (Ruggiero 1992). Furthermore, "while it is true that [for example] the Andean countries are coca producers and the United States and Europe are cocaine users, it is also true that the latter are producers of synthetic drugs and of the products needed for coca refining [acids]" (Sciacchitano 1991: 221). In one sense, therefore, while the west certainly experiences its own drug problems, it also continues to export such problems. However, this is a hidden and unacknowledged consequence of the development and profiteering of the western drug economy.

Cross-border trafficking, smuggling and crime

As the regional sources of origin of plant drugs change so do the modern trafficking routes. Hartnoll (1989: 43) summarizes:

> international trafficking routes are continually shifting according to the groups involved, international air connections, legitimate trade routes, political circumstances, law enforcement efforts, and so on. (For example) heroin is often routed indirectly via one or more transit countries in order to conceal its origin in known producer countries. Over recent years, Thailand has provided the main conduit for SE Asian heroin, mostly from Burma, that reaches the international market via Bangkok, Hong Kong, Indonesia, Singapore, and so on. The Indian sub-continent is a major outlet for SW Asian heroin, though overland routes through Iran, Turkey, the Balkans, or other Mediterranean countries are alternatives.

Boseley (1993) provides an example employing stages of the latter routes: "On January 9th 1993, a Panamanian-registered cargo ship owned by the Turkish mafia was intercepted in the Suez canal, carrying 14 tonnes of pure heroin from Afghanistan, via Pakistan.

The drugs with a street value of $14 billion (about £10 billion), were bound for Turkey and then on to Cyprus, Italy, Spain and the Netherlands. From there, they would be smuggled into the United Kingdom, Germany and France." Soggiu (1991: 382) describes the routes that cocaine trafficking may take through the Mediterranean and North Africa region, including the new and increasing significance of destabilized areas such as Lebanon. The Balkan region has also seen some destabilization recently but, from the traffickers point of view, social and political disruption actually have advantages and will probably have far more negative impact on the co-ordination of enforcement efforts. Unsurprisingly then, recent reports emphasize the continued importance of the "Balkan routes". In 1990, over half the heroin detected by Customs at points of entry into Britain had followed these routes and they remain key arteries for cross-Europe trafficking (Druglink 1991: 6). In November 1993, for example, British Customs made one of their biggest seizures ever, after tracking a lorry carrying 200 kilos of heroin concealed in a shipment of tomatoes, which had travelled from Turkey via this route (Campbell 1993). However, where the fighting in the region does threaten passage, supplies have simply been diverted through the Caucasus (Boseley 1993).

Transportation of drugs can also have an impact on transit countries apart from the final end-importer country: thus while drugs shipped through a transit country may be destined for a major consumer such as the US or parts of western Europe, there is a possibility that some of the drugs on the move will "spill over" into local markets (Hartnoll 1989). This appears to be the case with Greece and the former Yugoslavia – although on the other hand, such "spillover" may not occur in some locations where it might have been expected (for example, Austria, or parts of eastern Europe where drug markets have not developed until recently, and/or where currency has not been convertible).

As should be evident, drug trafficking through European territories is a cross-border crime *par excellence*, yet neither trafficking and smuggling nor cross-border crime generally, seem to have attracted much criminological attention (Van Duyne & Levi 1991). This may be changing but the literature remains sparse, with even recent comparisons between organized crime in western Europe and

America offering little comment on cross-national criminal organization in Europe (e.g. Fijnaut 1990) and reviews of "illicit drugs and organized crime" in Europe concentrating on enforcement issues to the surprising neglect of trafficking *per se* (Flood 1991, but see Savona et al. 1994 and Ruggiero 1994).

Smuggling

The degree of sophistication and innovation that goes into concealing drug shipments is, of course, by no means new (e.g. Fish 1962) and is undoubtedly simply an extension of the efforts to conceal contraband that have been made as long as morality and laws have forbidden things and taxes have made them expensive.

The strategies, techniques and arrangements employed in smuggling across European (and other, external) borders range from the obvious and ordinary – but not necessarily unsuccessful – to the highly innovative and unusual. To give a few established, but perhaps less well known examples:

Groups that have access to vehicles, legitimate retail outlets and good reason to engage in regular import–export business are particularly well placed to engage in smuggling operations. One respondent (who had been involved in smuggling drugs for Hells Angels groups and who is currently in a British prison for related offences) described one example of importation into the UK: "They [the drugs] can be transshipped in bike parts, frames etc. – you can get fourteen ounces of any powder [e.g. cocaine, heroin] into a frame." The drugs are then forwarded to bike and vehicle dealers who have a perfectly legitimate front business. The operators of these "fronts" may or may not be centrally involved in the importation operation but will naturally benefit financially. As such shipments may be recurrent but not too frequent, risks can be minimized. Our respondent continues:

> The drugs are put in like a heat sealed roll – you've seen the cling-film type things? Well, they're wrapped in separate parcels and then laid on a machine and rolled. It's like black plastic that seals them in and then they go inside the frames . . . All you do in the end is really, just chop the head-yoke off, tip it upside down and out comes your par-

cel. The frames are put together in Amsterdam or they're put together in America – usually for coke if it's coming from America. The weed [cannabis] all comes up through Europe – usually through Germany . . . cocaine comes through Spain.

Several respondents also pointed to the growth of the European and international mail system as vulnerable to smuggling operations. A cannabis dealer in Hammersmith, London, rightly observed that "It used to be really unusual to get letters from abroad – you know, when I was a kid it was only when the school gave you a pen-friend – now everyone knows people abroad, people live abroad, have houses there, retire there, relations, friends and so on – so there's birthdays, Christmas, parcels, letters etc." This small-scale dealer, operating quite independently, used European contacts and private box numbers to import small but profitable amounts of cannabis, and sometimes other drugs. Another informant, operating on a larger scale, observed that technology and mechanization of the mails had improved security in some ways but that the sheer bulk of mail meant that – as with the trafficking ploy of sending several couriers on a plane flight with the expectation that most will get through – sending several parcels or envelopes means most will be undetected:

Acid . . . comes from Amsterdam, very cheap. Sometimes it's just sent – there's certain ways of sending things through the post which can't be detected as long as they're slim envelopes and they're nothing too big. You know what I mean, you can send a thousand trips in a birthday card. They're bought for a guilder a piece in Amsterdam and sold here for £5, so just a thousand trips [units of acid impregnated paper] is enough to start your own business.

Other smuggling methods involve more elaborate conspiracies and organization, such as ownership or use of intercontinental trucks, with reputable clients and legal loads, but the capacity to hide drugs somewhere within the vehicle. Our Hell's Angel informant described how:

Lorry batteries were used at one time, where the lorry would go abroad, the driver would have his movements watched all the time so he's got his alibi. Sometime during the night, the batteries were taken off his wagon. What they were doing was they were driving them to the ferry port, leaving them there [the driver would go away] and the batteries were being changed. Well, what they were doing was they were taking the lorry batteries apart, cutting the cells in half, welding a plastic thing in the bottom, they're not the batteries you can see through, not like the white plastic ones, . . . two kilos [of heroin] put in the bottom, heat sealed in, re-acid [i.e. replace the acid]. Now that battery will start your wagon, as long as it's got a cooler unit on the back you've got enough power to take it on a ferry, take it off . . . Comes off at Dover, goes as far as Sandwich or Deal, goes into a garage and has his battery swopped.

For the Netherlands, Van Duyne & Levi (1991: 17) record a similar example: "some marijuana dealers entered the 'black' meat industry with a starting capital from their drugs enterprise. Some continued their drugs trafficking activities next to their upperworld meat trade; the frozen food transports have the advantage that drugs can be concealed in a way that is difficult to detect them by means of the trained 'sniffer dog'."

A different set of methods, employing legitimate travellers as unwitting but highly effective smugglers, was also described to us:

You've got groups [of smugglers] abroad, who pick on Dormobiles [and similar vehicles] that go round France and campsites, and when [the drivers/families] go off to the local pub at night and leave their Caravanette, a kilo's put in their spare-wheel. I mean, if they get a puncture and put the spare wheel on – tough shit – they've lost the gear, but it's nothing to them. . . .

[Where the drugs travel undiscovered –]

You just wait until it comes back to this country. Remember, at every foreign camp-site you have to give your registration papers, it's got your home address and everything, your vacation period, how long you're staying – are you with me? You just phone it through to the other end, you say "they're coming back on Thursday and they might spend a couple of nights on the south coast, but they'll be back for the weekend, the kids have got to go to school on Monday . . . Here's the address, blah, blah, blah. He drives a white Vauxhall, as well, so he'll be taking that to work and this [the caravanette or whatever] will probably be sat in his driveway or in his garage." A couple of guys go round and collect it. It's just a dead easy way [to smuggle].

Police respondents noted a related and now well known smuggling strategy which involves "setting up" a dummy or "real" smuggler. There are various permutations but this may be either an accomplice who fits the target-profiles of Customs inspectors and police but is in fact clean, or a travelling individual or group, such as the family holidaymakers described above, who in this case have a *small* amount of drugs unwittingly planted on their vehicle. Information is then passed to Customs and police anonymously in the expectation that they will concentrate their attention on the identified targets thus creating a diversion for the real, large-scale shipment going through at the same time.

Trafficking to European markets

(i) Heroin – an overview

In Chapter 5, we describe the development of heroin (and other drug) smuggling which has supplied the market in Turin. This is a path from amateur and co-operative ventures to diversified and organized enterprises. A similar path of development can be traced for the drug markets of most other western European countries, (for some examples of smuggling into Britain, see Dorn et al. 1992b). By the mid–late 1970s the trafficking of heroin and other drugs had become a major and organized international business.

Trafficking routes are strongly influenced by geo-political factors. From the Indian subcontinent, overland smuggling of heroin by truck or car still takes place through the Balkan region. As noted earlier, the importance of this route has long been established but its renewed significance reflects recent shifts in military and political spheres: thus, "the route begins by taking advantage of the end of the Soviet presence in Afghanistan, then crosses Iran, now free of the war with Iraq. Lorries are loaded in Turkey and enter Europe in Bulgaria" (Druglink 1991: 6). Thereafter all European countries are relatively accessible. To reach the UK, Germany and Belgium are the main countries crossed, but the domestic markets of Germany, the Netherlands, France and other European countries, are equally accessible by this route.

(ii) cocaine – an overview

Obviously, South American connections are involved at some point – though where this involvement ends and European claims begin differs in different circumstances and countries. There have been numerous reports of attempts by Columbian traffickers to establish themselves in European centres while others argue that South American traffickers must now target Europe because the US market has reached a saturation point. This argument seems dubious given the vastly different levels of use across North America but one does not have to agree with this view to accept that cocaine will be increasingly available in the 1990s. INCB figures for 1986 indicated that 1.4 tons were seized in Europe in 1986, an 80 per cent increase on 1985 (Lewis 1989: 36, INCB 1987); since the mid 1980s reports of seizures from member countries of Interpol to its General Secretariat have risen rapidly: in 1987 – 2.4 tons; in 1988 – 5.3 tons; in 1989 – 6 tons; and in 1990 – 13 tons: representing an increase over 1985 of nearly 1500 per cent (Kendall 1991: 398). UK Customs seizure figures for 1990 indicate a continued upward trend in cocaine smuggling with Columbia the "largest single source" and evidence of a "growing secondary route from Jamaica and the Eastern seaboard of America – primarily female couriers bringing in kilo amounts" (Druglink 1991: 6).

The main points of entry into Europe are Madrid, Lisbon, Amsterdam, Frankfurt and Copenhagen. Spain, Portugal, and to some degree, Italy, have long established ties with South America (Lewis 1989: 36, Stewart-Clarke 1986). Importation of cocaine to individual European countries may be conducted by independent local groups who manage to establish links with South American producers and refiners. However, the cocaine business can also be a multi-national enterprise of major proportions. This was recently illustrated by "Operation Green Ice", which was based on two years of investigation work and culminated in about 200 arrests in eight countries and the seizure of $65 million in assets. Professional criminals were arrested in Spain, Italy, Costa Rica, Columbia, and Canada, while money launderers were arrested in the UK and Switzerland, and a "financial adviser" in the Netherlands (Tisdall & Vulliamy 1992, D'Avanzo 1992). It must be said, however, as this book and the work of others (e.g. Dorn et al. 1992b, Savona et al. 1994) suggest, that such multinational conspiracies and enterprises are rare.

There are also reports that Columbian exporters had established business fronts in, and supply routes to, the eastern Bloc – and from there to western Europe – even before political change. For example, a joint Czech-Columbia venture to ship sugar, rice and soya to Czechoslovakia was set up in 1989. This operation was used to smuggle cocaine destined for western Europe (Davies 1992). In 1991, police say that 440 lbs of cocaine were seized in Bohemia and at Gdansk in Poland, which would ultimately have been smuggled onward to the Netherlands and Britain (ibid.).

Distributing drugs in European Markets

Post-importation, Lewis (1989) argues that cocaine trading techniques in Europe are similar in essence to those described by Adler (1985) in her case study on California's west coast: "importers sell multiple kilos to . . . bulk buyers, who in turn re-sell at a straightforward mark-up or, through dilution, at a concealed mark-up. Kilos are divided into quarter-kilo or half kilo units and, thence, into ounces or their rough equivalent in grams. Distribution chains seem neither as extenuated as heroin delivery systems, nor as diffuse at retail level (Preble & Casey 1969, Lewis et al. 1985)" (Lewis 1989: 37). Major importation and large scale sale of both cannabis and cocaine in Europe are now "effectively dominated by coalitions of professional criminals or import-export traders who move drugs along with legitimate merchandise . . ." (ibid.).

In a more recent review, Lewis (1994) has offered a broad-brush description of some characteristics of heroin distribution, retailing and markets in western Europe between 1970 and 1990:

> Retail heroin was dealt initially in the centres of major cities. In due course dealing extended beyond the centres and beyond the cities themselves. This "shift to the periphery" in which activity radiated outwards to the suburbs, (particularly those districts displaying high indices of social deprivation) was evident in Paris by 1978 . . . and in Rome by 1980 . . . (ibid.: 43)

In general terms, the heroin market expanded across Europe in the 1980s, although as Lewis (ibid.) remarks, a European decline in overdose deaths, along with a fall in seizures, "raised hopes that consumption might have peaked in 1986". This was not the case, however, and overdoses rose again in the late 1980s, partly attributed to increased purity levels.

Based on research from Britain, Italy and other European countries, Lewis suggests the following "approximate" levels in drug markets: a) importers and importer combinations; b) distributors; c) small-scale wholesalers and apartment dealers; d) retail sales – street and appointment dealers, e) network suppliers and user-sellers; f) end-users and street consumers.

Other models of the drug market identify different ideal-type participants which might be complementary to or fruitfully combined with Lewis's to illustrate the fluidity and complexity of the market (Dorn & South 1990, Dorn et al. 1992b: see below).

At the bottom of the hierarchy of participants in drug markets are the end-users and street consumers. These may be the most visible and vulnerable to enforcement attentions as well as the other social problems that can accompany heavy drug use:

> "Historic" public dealing venues such as Piccadilly in central London, the Dam in Amsterdam, the Zoo in Berlin and the Parco Lambro in Milan tend to be places where i) casual users or young initiates, unfamiliar with the market, come to buy; ii) old-style street survivors congregate, partly to stay in touch and, partly, in the hope of obtaining drugs or cash by interposing themselves between retail dealers

and potential customers; iii) regular consumers, whose usual points of supply have been lost or terminated, seek a temporary substitute. Quality is usually lower, prices higher, weights shorter, and theft and fraud more frequent in such a context. "Birds of passage", surviving on the social fringes of a host country, are able to work as suppliers in such high profile locations because of their very transience. They are vulnerable as single individuals but, because of their impermanence, the dealing in which they engage is less subject to systematic police and monopolistic criminal pressure. (ibid.: 52)

Some dimensions of trafficking, markets and crime in individual countries

Case study countries 1: Britain

Dorn & South (1990) present a typology of possible participants in the drug market in Britain and have subsequently (Dorn et al. 1992b) modified this description, providing case histories. The categories developed generally relate to established "types" described elsewhere in the empirical literature; other researchers have employed categories of the typology in their own analyses of local drug markets (e.g. Fraser & George 1988). We do not apply this typology here in any strict or rigorous sense, indeed the deficiencies of such static models when applied to situations of fluidity and change such as drug markets, were noted by the original authors. However, we shall refer to some of these types and, therefore, describe them briefly:

1. *Trading charities* – enterprises involved in the drug business, because of ideological commitments to drugs (e.g. cannabis, ecstasy), with some profit being welcome but generally a secondary motive.

2. *Mutual societies* – friendship networks of user-dealers who support each other and sell or exchange drugs among themselves in a reciprocal fashion (in the Turin case study such characteristics are found among the early heroin user groups of the city).

3. *Sideliners* – originally defined in a pure sense, as the licit busi-

ness enterprise that begins to trade in drugs as an (occasional) sideline. However, "sidelining" is also a useful description of the activities of criminal organizations that "sideline" into licit economy activities, whether to launder and invest dirty money or to facilitate trafficking or both.

4. *Criminal diversifiers* – the existing criminal enterprise that diversifies its operations into the drugs economy; this may be on an occasional or regular basis.

5. *Opportunistic irregulars* – individuals or small groups who involve themselves in a variety of activities in the "irregular economy", including drug dealing.

6. *Retail specialists* – enterprises reflecting a clear division of labour, with a manager employing people in a variety of specialized rôles to distribute drugs to users, from street level upwards. (Dorn et al. 1992b: xiii).

At the level of significance for European trade, it is largely the professional criminal diversifiers and the legitimate/semi-legitimate sidelining businesses (such as import/export firms) that should be noted.

For London, Lewis (1989: 42) argues that the involvement of professional criminal firms started in the mid 1970s with importation by TIR truck and boat, of ton shipments of cannabis. Given the profit to be made in the drugs business, the step to importation and distribution of heroin and cocaine was a short one (ibid.: 43).

It is during the late 1970s and early 1980s, that the British illegal drug market developed significantly, in terms of size, diversity, serious criminal involvement and corresponding enforcement response. Burr's (1983a,b) ethnographic research in the Piccadilly Circus area (the Dilly) of London, found that the leading product on sale for a relatively long period had been physeptone. Other prescribed drugs were also available. The Piccadilly clientele was partly formed by street users without reliable dealer contacts, who therefore had to run the high risk of apprehension in an area with constant police activity directed at the pornography business, prostitutes, kerb crawlers, drunks and drug dealers. What is important to note is that the market for pharmaceutical opiates, in Piccadilly and elsewhere, played an important rôle in facilitating the subsequent (and perhaps the parallel) circulation of illicitly imported drugs. The grey market which developed through the 1960s and 1970s forged expertise and structures which proved of crucial importance in the later distribution of other illegal drugs.

In Britain and other European countries during the 1960s and early 1970s, small-scale dealing and distribution principally involved groups banding together to purchase drugs on some mutual benefit basis, or individuals who were themselves user/dealers and who made a small profit from regular supply to a relatively small circle or set of groups (the mutual societies and trading charities described earlier). At this level of distribution little professionalism was evident or required. More sophisticated and complex participants, such as non-users/distributors, were almost absent. However, in the late 1970s, the presence of small-scale criminal entrepreneurs who occasionally entered the market was observed in some areas of London. These individuals or groups were not associated with the drug scene and did not use the substances they sold (although unlike earlier generations of professional criminals they may have had some experience with illegal drugs such as amphetamine and cannabis in the 1960s; Lewis 1989: 42). These groups engaged in stealing pharmaceuticals from chemist shops or from chemical warehouses. They rarely resorted to retail selling, but preferred supplying small-scale distributors.

It is hard to assess the extent to which the maintenance-prescribing policy of the 1960s favoured the spread of heroin use and growth of the market in London or elsewhere. Some commentators are inclined to think that "the increase was directly related to the new regulations of 1968. As supplies of legal heroin declined, so the illicit market escalated . . ." (Leech 1991: 54). By the late 1970s, a new recreational heroin culture had developed which was largely unfamiliar to older users and mainly involved the young (Royal College of Psychiatrists 1987). In the accounts of some older heroin users, the new users were seen as being indiscriminate in resorting both to the grey market of pharmaceutical heroin and the illegal market. One ex-user described such behaviour:

> The youths would pursue the "scripters" and try to get some pure heroin, but if they didn't succeed in that, they would buy the No. 3 from the Chinese. The Chinese had never "pushed" heroin, they traditionally used it in their circles as a recreational substance. They eventually turned

into "pushers" when a new generation of users "pushed" them to do so, and when they realized the commercial value of the substance.

It is well known that heroin from non-pharmaceutical sources had been available in Britain since the early 1960s. Its use seems to have been principally (though not exclusively) confined to the Chinese community. In this milieu, heroin was mainly inhaled for recreational purposes. With the decline of the availability of prescribed heroin, the price of the Chinese powder increased considerably. At the same time, the price of prescribed heroin still available on the market rose by 300 per cent: in the early 1970s, the cost of one grain reaching £3 (Hartnoll & Mitcheson et al. 1980). This trend went hand in hand with the official establishment of methadone treatment programmes, which were often rejected by the new users. Methadone was more acceptable to users if it was provided in injectable form, whereas the syrup that was increasingly prescribed had to be taken orally and proved widely unpopular. For injectors then, heroin (either illegally imported or pharmaceutical) remained the favourite substance on the market.

It is impossible to say with certainty how the subsequent dynamics of the market were stimulated, but during the late 1970s an increase in demand for heroin coincided with a simultaneous increase in supply. On balance, it is perhaps this latter factor and the sheer availability of heroin that led to rapid escalation of use. This increase in supply can be related to three factors: first, higher levels of production; secondly, the widening of distribution networks internationally; and finally the emergence of a number of European centres as crucial transshipment points (Lewis et al. 1985). The period around 1978-9 was a critical phase for the spread of heroin in Britain and London in particular. The Thai variety suddenly disappeared (perhaps due to crop failure in the Golden Triangle, or successful police and customs operations) and many users turned instead to the Iranian variety. For several reasons this was now available in large quantities: "Political events in Iran itself [had] contributed to a substantial increase in supply on the British market" (ibid.: 282) and the overthrow of the Shah in 1979 led to exiles converting capital with a resulting dramatic increase in the amount of heroin available on the street. Burr (1984: 338) records that "immediately after the Iranian revolution, the Kensington, Notting Hill and Chelsea areas, where many Iranians settled, became for a time the major foci of non-pharmaceutical heroin dealing in London". Of crucial importance was that the Iranian heroin could be smoked. Such heroin allegedly continued to feed the London market for about two years after the collapse of the old Iranian regime, imported by some of the new settlers who availed themselves of well established connections with wholesale distributors in their home country.

According to Burr (1984) this new heroin market could be described as elitist: visitors from Europe, living in prestigious parts of Kensington, purchased drugs weekly as if shopping in up-market boutiques. However, other researchers described Iranian heroin as being crudely refined and hence privileged users who could afford it avoided Iranian heroin and instead sought pharmaceutical or white, Southeast Asian No. 4 heroin, a much-valued variety. At this time pharmaceutical heroin was retailing for as much as £110 per gram in the summer of 1981 and so-called "Thai" for £120 in spring of the same year (Lewis et al. 1985: 286). These prices were sufficiently low, relatively speaking, to mean that users were presented with a reasonable range of choice: when the Iranian variety flooded the market, prices declined in all areas of London. Choice of areas where heroin could be purchased and dealers to buy from widened, and conditions were right for the spread of non-injecting heroin use across social classes (Pearson et al. 1987).

To summarize, the increased availability of heroin at the end of the 1970s and in the early 1980s, was accompanied by differentiation among users and a broadening of their social characteristics. New heroin cultures sprang up which were more compatible with diverse lifestyles. In this sense, smokable Iranian heroin played an important rôle: it had made heroin accessible to those who did not identify themselves with the "junkie" image, and did not see heroin as a symbol of marginalization or self-exclusion (Ruggiero 1992). Indeed, for some of the new heroin users, the drug was assimilated into a "normal" lifestyle of deviant behaviour, risk, profit and recreational reward (Auld et al. 1986). Both an elitist and a mass commodity, heroin could now also be administered according to taste, status and self-image. Iranian heroin could be smoked, but after rudimentary acidification, it could also be injected. The key health and policy significance of this was that the easy smoking of the drug might later give way to injection (for various reasons – economy, peer pressure, experimental desire, and so on). Hence smoking heroin drew more users into the pool of potential intravenous injectors who were at risk of HIV infection. More specifically, Ruggiero (1992: 75) draws attention to the way that a decline in purity, after heroin has passed along the distribution chain, may also encourage a shift from smoking to intravenous use.

By 1982 the presence of Pakistani heroin on the market had become prominent (Customs and Excise 1983) and the prevalence of this new product made the previous distinctions between types of heroin based on national origin less relevant (Henman et al. 1985). Heroin became an increasingly versatile commodity, its country of production no longer constituting a label for quality. Quality was simply identified with its perceived potency and determined by purity. Researchers in London observed that the wholesale price of heroin in 1983 was lower than it had been in 1980, falling by 20 per cent in relation to inflation (Lewis et al. 1985).

Overall, the shift from pharmaceutical to Chinese heroin, and from this to Iranian and Pakistani heroin, marked a parallel shift both in the cultures of use and in the characteristics of heroin itself. This shift was also consistent with the market modifications that occurred, both in the nature of demand and in the nature of availability and dealing. The bohemian culture of the early 1960s, initially associated with illicit users of pharmaceutical heroin, was then taken up by the users of Chinese heroin. By contrast, the subsequent users of Iranian and Pakistani heroin in the late 1970s and early 1980s, did not need or seek to embrace any "countercultural" values. If we can speak of a heroin epidemic occurring in London, Merseyside, and elsewhere in England and Scotland in the 1980s, this was due not only to the increase in availability but also to the changing nature of the opiates available and the changing expectations of users (Pearson et al. 1987, Giggs 1991; for a cautious view of the "epidemic" analogy, see Young 1987: 426–8).

Of course, another factor influencing the shape of the heroin market was the emergence of, and frequent merger with, other drug markets: "participants in [heroin and cocaine distribution systems] often overlap, and consumption, hence diversion, occurs at all levels, wholesale and retail, oligopolistic and competitive" (Lewis

1989: 44). Since its emergence in the 1970s, the London cocaine market has involved various groups – freelance interests, South American importers and British professional crime groups. According to Lewis (1989: 43)

> In 1982 intelligence reports suggested that cocaine trafficking in the United Kingdom was dominated by Britons, as opposed to some other recipient countries where non-native groups, particularly South Americans, had established themselves (Drug Enforcement Administration 1982). The informal nature of much of the British market and the social conservatism and reserve of its participants may have encouraged this; South American groups sometimes find it difficult to forge links with British groups capable of purchasing and distributing bulk consignments in the same way that British criminals initially found it hard to move into the cannabis market in the early 1970s.

In Chapter 4 we shall bring our description of the London heroin and polydrug use scene up to date.

Case study country 2: Italy

According to a number of researchers, current patterns of drug use in Italy reflect several values dominant in Italian society. On the one hand, drug use is deemed to be consistent with a prevailing culture of hedonism in which people value short-term pleasures and have little regard for long term goals. On the other hand, drug use is seen as an expression of the dominant medico-pharmaceutic culture which, for years, has promised remedies against fatigue and pain, and panaceas against distress of varied degrees. Unsurprisingly however, such broad claims cannot be applied across the board. In Naples, for example, hedonistic values can only partly explain the dramatic diffusion of heroin use. Here, the phenomenon is related to various traditional factors which characterize the social structure of the city. These factors include – the existence of wide-spread illegality or semi-legality in some sectors of the local economy, the previous vivacity of a distribution network supplying both licit and illicit commodities, and the presence of organized crime endowed with previously accumulated capital and capable of recruiting a large criminal labour-force (Ruggiero 1992, Ruggiero & Vass 1992).

Nor does such an analysis seem applicable in a context such as Milan. One illuminating study in this city, based on interviews with a sample of petty property offenders, found that many rejected the prospect of taking either a legitimate job or employment by organized crime on a regular basis (Bianchi 1986). They likened organized crime to ordinary systems of employment, both being regarded as "brutal exploiters". Some showed a sense of pride in their illegal "professionality" and independence, and claimed to be unprepared to relinquish either in exchange for a "secure" job in an organized group. Research conducted in Bologna in the mid 1970s (Faccioli & Quargnolo 1987) found that among young heroin distributors in the city only some shared a background in an identifiable criminal subculture. This led the researchers to give up any attempt to investigate causal connections between social, economic and cultural variables and drug use and distribution. The utilization of a control-group, comprised of "normal" youths, revealed the existence of many common elements shared with young heroin addicts: a sense of personal crisis, the search for identity, affective disenchantment, uncertainty about the future, lack of status, etc. Other studies in Italy report that prior involvement in a criminal subculture was very difficult to find even among middle- and high-rank heroin distributors. Examining the case of Verona, Arlacchi & Lewis (1989) concluded that the diffusion of hard drugs took place within the structure of the local, highly efficient, *licit* economy. We shall expand upon this important point later, in Chapter 5.

Nonetheless, drug markets and availability in Italy can hardly be analyzed without reference to organized crime. While rooted in traditional cultures and criminal activities, organized crime has found drugs enterprises to be an unanticipated spur to development. In Italy, at the lowest levels of distribution and consumption, heroin as a commodity is associated with extremely dispersed forms of crime. At the highest levels of processing and distribution, however, heroin is a commodity associated with highly structured forms of crime. Such a situation was anticipated more than two decades ago, when it was hypothesized that the thriving illicit cigarette distribution network would soon be converted to serve the distribution of heroin

(Pantaleone 1966). Confirmation of this trend was offered by subsequent research which produced evidence that the finances accumulated in cigarette smuggling were being reinvested in hard drugs by both the mafia and the Neapolitan network of organized crime, the camorra (Pizzorno & Arlacchi 1985, Flosi 1988, Ruggiero 1993d). Heroin was the lever which also allowed organized crime groups to expand their intervention into legal activities. According to some Sicilian judges, in the early 1980s part of the drugs market proceeds was invested

> in the building business, in agriculture, [and] in licit industrial and commercial activities . . . Palermo is probably the Italian town with the highest number of building sites, it is the only urban centre where, despite the economic crisis, new luxurious shops keep flourishing. It could be estimated that a fourth of the economy of the town is sustained by the production and distribution of heroin (Chinnici & Mannino 1983).

Until relatively recently in Italy, it was quite commonly argued that the mafia and the camorra were "residual phenomena" that were destined to disappear as the process of modernization proceeded. This has indeed proved to be a short-sighted view (Enzensberger 1979). Instead, the move into drug markets has contributed to the parallel modernization of organized crime as it developed entrepreneurial skills that could be utilized in both illicit and licit business (Arlacchi 1983, Catanzaro 1988) – a development with similarities in other parts of Europe and North America.

A clearer picture of such entrepreneurial skills emerges when we consider the economic cycle through which heroin as a commodity will proceed: the production and the transformation of raw material; the operations of import, export and transit of the final product; the warehousing and distribution; the activities connected to money-laundering, which in turn, according to Judge Carlo Palermo "are connected to illicit trafficking of money, sometimes of a licit origin, and intermingled with smuggling of jewels and arms" (Palermo 1983: 32). Another Judge, Vito Zincani has emphasized that the reinvestment of the proceeds of drug dealing and trafficking is of great interest if we wish to identify the features of contemporary organized crime. These reinvestments confer to organized crime enough economic and political power to thrive in the very heart of the legal society, and to control a part of the vital sectors of its economy (Zincani 1989).

Overall, the literature regarding the relationship between organized crime and drugs in Italy is very large and suggests several conclusions. The growth of availability and use of hard drugs has favoured more organizational efficiency in the criminal groups already in existence. It has also encouraged the formation of new organized groups which are as structured as their traditional counterparts. Research also suggests that drug distribution promotes some tendencies towards a monopoly situation where one criminal group attempts to prevail over others. However, if the category "monopoly" is considered as a characteristic involving exclusive control of the markets by means of violence, this characteristic is not the most relevant attribute of the Sicilian mafia. As already noted, many researchers share the opinion that the strength of the mafia today is to be found more in its legal rather than in its illegal performances. Furthermore, the cost of suppressing competition is increasingly rising both in terms of the use of violence and in terms of arranging political corruption. Competition therefore persists, fragmentation of the market is characteristic, flux is the norm. The illegal markets, therefore, seem populated by small firms, some of which are peripheral and ephemeral, in a highly mobile and active scenario (Reuter 1984, Dorn & South 1990).

Following from this observation, we might argue that the term "disorganized crime" (Reuter 1984) may be more appropriate when discussing heroin markets on a local basis. These seem to be animated by small or middle-range firms which cohabit, or alternatively shift into a leading position only for a limited time and in circumscribed territories. Several sources of evidence confirm this. Judge Falcone's investigation proved that decisions regarding the involvement of the mafia in illegal drug business transactions were not taken by some central body. Rather, *initially* they were the result of personal and group initiatives (Falcone 1991). All supergrasses informing on the mafia confirmed that the original finances invested in drugs enterprises came from neither common organizational assets nor the collective wealth of particular mafia families. Instead the money invested was put up by individuals. Members of traditional Italian organized crime who resolved to enter the drug business, therefore had a new opportunity to build partnerships with other investors from outside their "family" and indeed from outside the mafia (Arlacchi 1992b, Gambetta 1992). Increasingly, therefore, it has been possible for members of traditional organized crime groups who became active in the drug economy, to partially sever links with their "family" and the overall organization to which they had belonged – although, of course, over time, traditional crime organizations (mafia, etc.) have also moved into the drugs business to become key players. Significantly, however, none of these groups have managed to establish a monopoly over the distribution of illegal drugs. Rather, among large operators, conditions of oligopolistic competition tend to prevail in the national and specific local markets they service, while medium and lower level distributors compete in less stable and fragmentary markets.

For successful drugs enterprises and their investors there is no shortage of other fields of activity into which they can diversify as legitimate enterprises, operating on a national and/or international scale:

> The enormous financial capacity of the mafia determines a process of gradual overlapping between the criminal and the legal economies . . . and it fosters a logic which is very similar to the normal logic of development. This entails that all forms of enterprise are taken into account by the criminal groups, including the more advanced forms of production (Galante 1986: 120–21).

In Chapter 5, we shall provide a description and analysis of the heroin market in Torino which also takes into account the problems connected with the presence and nature of organized crime in the city. We shall also provide examples of other groups involved and of developments in distribution and trafficking related to this market.

Netherlands

The 1919 Opium Act made transporting and dealing in prohibited drugs an offence in the Netherlands. However, this did not prevent the development of what De Kort & Korf (1992: 133) call "a massive smuggling traffic". There were three dimensions to this traffic: first, a sizeable semi-legal trade in which large pharmaceutical firms and others exported large shipments of drugs to China and the USA, circumventing the law or exploiting loopholes – "legally produced substances thus found their way into the illegal circuit via a detour" (ibid.: 134). Secondly, opium was illegally imported, coming from Turkey to Marseille and on to Rotterdam and Amsterdam, and finding a market in the Chinese dock area communities. These communities had grown since port employers had brought in Chinese labour to break a seamen's strike in 1911 (ibid.: 136). Mirroring ways in which ethnic difference and drug use were linked and vilified elsewhere when labour market conditions changed and made them unwelcome, the Chinese were the group most frequently prosecuted after the 1919 Act (cf. Helmer 1975, Kohn 1992). The third trade was in cocaine, manufactured by German companies such as Boerhringer & Merck, then smuggled across German and Belgian borders to the Netherlands, Belgium and France.

Police opinion is that opiate dealing was controlled by the Chinese Triads until the end of the 1970s, after which the market opened up and today it is Turkish, Moroccan and Pakistani syndicates which predominate (De Kort & Korf 1992: 140). This official view and the implications drawn are important – and we shall have more to say on this issue later, in our analysis of the significance of race and racism in the division of labour operating within the London drug market (Chapter 4). As De Kort & Korf (1992: 140–41) argue:

> In other countries, drug dealers are likewise seen to belong mostly to ethnic minorities. That aliens and immigrants take part in the drug trade is certainly not to be denied. In view of their generally low status in Western society, and their social ties with drug producing and transit countries, their participation would indeed seem self-evident. But that falls short of justifying the conclusion that they are the main culprits in the current drug problems confronting the West. (cf. Dorn & South 1984, Auld et al. 1984).

Regarding the structure of drug-crime and trafficking operations in the Netherlands, Van Duyne & Levi (1991) report research on 19 drug trafficking enterprises. Here, and reflecting aspects of the drug/crime market in Britain and Italy,

> the operations of the small and medium scale drugs-enterprise, including the handling of the profits, are typically an underground economy and have no direct relations to the "upperworld": legitimate industry or the bureaucracies of the state. However, this changes when the crime enterprise expands the volume of its trade. The contraband can no longer be smuggled in small packets tied to the body of the courier or carried in prepared suitcases. The thousands of kilos of marijuana must be hidden in ships or lorries, which implies that the crime enterprise has to make capital goods investments. These are registered in official register offices, which can render the criminal enterprise visible to law enforcement agencies. This implies that the crime enterprise will need "legal front" companies, to which these capital goods can be registered. In this way he enters the upperworld-economy. (ibid.: 12)

Illicit money management requires the services of the legitimate financial sectors once funds generated are too large for expenditure, loss or absorption within the cash based underground or irregular economy. Money surpluses are most easily spent or moved "legally" through the creation of legal companies or use of legal commercial services which will re-invest money, in other words through "entering the financial secrecy industry" (ibid.: 12–19, Walter 1989, South 1992). Establishing legal fronts with limited liability and using the professional services of lawyers and other advisors can be relatively straightforward or involve a complex picture of transfers and cross-transfers. A case described by Van Duyne & Levi (1991: 20) is illustrative:

> Two big dealers in hashish and cocaine (brothers) owned five textile and leather shops, two shell companies and three firms for electronic equipment, financed by a holding company. Between these firms an extensive and complex flow of money was created involving Gibralter, Switzerland and Luxembourg. The enterprise was advised by two ex-

perts for foreign money transfers and two legal advisers for
the creation of legal bodies. Of course the names of the two
brothers did not appear on the list of shareholders. The
shares were in the possession of the girlfriend of one of
them.

Van Duyne & Levi (ibid.) usefully contrast the drug trafficking
enterprise with other forms of entrepreneurial crime by drawing attention to the fact that the latter may need to create "upperworld"
legal companies in order to "make victims and profits" whereas the
former principally needs such fronts to facilitate the movement of
its commodity and its profits:

> as long as the drugs enterprise pays its bills and taxes it will
> not go bankrupt and its legal front will draw no attention
> from law enforcement agencies. Some of the smartest drugs
> traffickers are aware of this and their legal front companies
> are just part of the legitimate industry using the legal cargo
> to hide the illegal import or export only. (The Colombian
> cocaine enterprises appear to have found a very smart mix
> of legal and illegal businesses, the legal ones ranging from
> fruit companies to shoe repair firms). As the threat comes
> usually only from the police and competitors who may steal
> the contraband (or be informants to the police) and not
> from creditors, the drugs enterprise (including the legal
> front company) may continue for years. (ibid.: 15)

As we shall indicate in the case studies below (Chapters 4 and 5),
there is here "a more intricate interaction with and penetration of
the legitimate industry than is accounted for by the simple and classical model of organized crime with its clear division of 'underworld' . . . and 'upperworld'" (ibid.: 16).

Criminal justice policy and drugs in the Netherlands
Up until 1965, the Amsterdam narcotics unit was comprised of just
two detectives. It was established after the Second World War to respond to the smuggling of drugs pilfered from the stores of the de-
feated German army and being trafficked along the border (De
Kort & Korf 1992: 137). Since then drug enforcement has ex-

panded, particularly in the 1980s. The larger municipal areas have specialist investigators and the Hague-based National Criminal Intelligence Service hosts the Central Narcotics Agency. Here intelligence with domestic or international significance is processed and passed to local police investigators or overseas liaison officers, or shared co-operatively with representatives of other countries' drug enforcement organizations. As elsewhere, the police face investigative difficulties in drugs cases for there are no complainants or victims of crime in the traditional sense. Hence, as De Kort & Korf (1992: 134–5) observe, "from an early date we witness the advent of crime fighting tactics which still today are not free from controversy. In 1922 it was already clear that without informers the police had a hopeless task." This remains the case today, with similar controversy attached to the employment of techniques such as "buy-bust" and "sell bust" in operations that may step over the mark to become cases of entrapment and invite condemnation of *agents provocateur* (Dorn, et al. 1992b, Ch. 8).

The state of the Dutch prison system reflects the fact that the Netherlands is not as lenient with drug offenders as its image has it (Mol & Trautmann 1991: 17). There is now a shortage of facilities and "prison building programmes are taking into account that, of the 2000 new cells [that were] to be completed in 1990, 1200 will have to be reserved for offenders under the Opium Act. The heavy burden imposed on the criminal justice system is illustrated by the fact that more than 30 per cent of all prisoners are addicted to drugs" (Samson 1990: 43). As with other prison systems in Europe it is clear that drug use within prisons is a significant problem and this has serious implications for the general health and HIV/AIDS status of prisoners.

Overall, Dutch policy assumes that the containment or prevention of drug supply is unlikely to be achieved in the near future but what can be successful is containment of demand if this aim is supported by an infrastructure encouraging social controls and offering health and welfare services etc. (Samson 1990: 44)

Germany

Youth cultures, bohemian nightlife, a location at the cross-roads of post-war Europe, indigenous criminal groups and a large and marginalized population of "Guestworkers" have all contributed to the development of drug markets in major German cities, such as Hamburg, Frankfurt and, of course, Berlin. Kreuzer et al. (1991a: 154) note that the early drug scene, up to the beginning of the 1970s, "was marked by decentralized types of drug procurement – any addict could get drugs cheaply by breaking into a pharmacy, forging prescriptions, or getting hold of them under false pretences. Later, a unified and complex (but not mafia-controlled) black market formed around the raw substance for the 'Berliner Tinke' (Heroin No. 1) and then increasingly for heroin itself."

The older drug market was principally organized around "soft" drugs and differed significantly from the new market for hard drugs in terms of dealing practices, profits to be made and channels of communication. The heroin market started in the west and moved eastward in Berlin between 1972 and 1974. Since then, Kreuzer et al. (ibid.) observe that the market and its structure have remained fairly unchanged and have been reproduced elsewhere (although unification may have had an impact these authors were not able to take into account). Other "public markets" for the sale of heroin and other drugs include:

> the "hash meadow" in Frankfurt, the *Kurfurstendamm* underground station in Berlin, the *Munchener Freiheit* in Munich, and the *Herrengarten* in Darmstadt. Anyone can get hold of drugs at such places as long as a few rules are observed. The dealers, go-betweens, and customers are subject to certain regulations that are defined by the market (amounts, prices, dealing practices, advertising, protection obligations). The social fabric of these scenes is very elastic and the police appear to have difficulty in penetrating it. Other public venues for drug sales are discotheques and all-night bars.

Interestingly, the researchers argue that for their respondents, participation in the market changed constantly and that "lasting success as a dealer was rare". We shall return to the point that it is actually quite difficult to really succeed as a dealer, in our case studies below.

Patterns of offences associated with involvement in the drug market are familiar. Users rely on legal income (earned, sick pay, social security etc.), but also commit a number of common crimes for money. These are generally simple, easily and quickly performed, requiring little or no skill, and repeated regularly. Kreuzer et al. (1991b: 412) report that the addicts in their studies "had committed a large number of different crimes in the course of their lives and in the previous year. With a few exceptions, they did not tend to specialize in a particular type of offence. Just as the 'multi-user' is the most commonly found consumer of drugs, the 'multi-delinquent' is the most commonly found criminal on the drug scene." Since the early 1970s, theft of drugs themselves has decreased significantly. In the study reported by Kreuzer et al. (1991a: 155) "about one-third of the subjects, and of these twice as many men as women, had had a history of delinquency prior to their drug career. In the other cases, either the drug and delinquency careers developed simultaneously or crime was resorted to in order to get money to pay for the drugs. Sooner or later, most users of hard drugs become known to the police." When drug users appear before the courts, women users seem to be treated more leniently than men, as are "dependent" as opposed to "criminal" drug users (ibid.: 156).

France

Ingold (1985a) provides an interesting description of heroin distribution in the drug market of Paris in the early 1980s. In this account, the market involves both large structured organizations as well as a number of small importers and traffickers and the distribution system is, by nature, shifting and haphazard:

> In theory, we can distinguish three levels: dealers who operate from their homes and sell to users, intermediaries and street peddlers; street peddlers who sell to users, and intermediaries whose only customers are users. However, in practice these distribution categories are in a state of constant flux, affected as they are by movements of drugs and funds. The whole system can also be affected by users' "plans" and "deals", the "plans" being their means of selling some of the amount they acquire on a one-off basis. These two factors must be borne in mind in any discussion of the three distribution levels and explain why transac-

93

tions are rapid, furtive and sometimes improvised (Ingold 1985a: 209).

However, going beyond a simple description of the distribution system, Ingold (ibid.: 212) also provides an analysis of the rule "structure" and economic entrapment which capture small-scale user-dealers within the drug economy:

> Because of its characteristic structure, the world of drug abuse becomes a specifically defined social "space" obeying a number of day-to-day unwritten rules – an insular phenomenon or, in other words, a space organized by "a rule" as the term is used by Jean Baudrillard (1979): "The rule is immanent to a restricted, limited system which it describes but does not transcend, and within this system it is immutable. It does not aim at universality and, strictly speaking, it has no external prolongation since it does not institute any internal separation."
>
> In this world, the circulation of funds resembles the sort of "pyramid" or "golden circle" swindle where each customer buys a fictitious share so as to create a fund and make the money in it circulate, the only beneficiaries being the people at the top of the pyramid or in the centre of the circle. This economic structure explains why the only hope for a user who gets caught up in it is to forge blindly ahead. And when he can no longer keep up the pace, he will have to start taking stock of his consumption, not in terms of money or heroin but in terms of what he has lost. It is by applying this concept of loss . . . that we can reach a deeper understanding of the extraordinary efficiency of the distribution process and the strange motives of users.

There are interesting suggestions raised here but unfortunately, we have not seen this analysis taken any further.

Eastern Europe

Poland

According to Watson (1991: 13) "The peculiarities of the opiate supply mechanisms in Poland go a long way towards explaining why supply has failed to create escalating demand" (so far . . .). As described earlier, the domestic opiate drug market is literally a home grown affair: the wide availability of the simple technology to turn equally available opium plant product into opiate drugs means that nearly all drug users are also, at some time if not all of the time, drug producers (ibid.). However, their processed produce is therefore often for own consumption and there have been other factors limiting the development of a large scale illegal market. This situation may now be changing with increased gangsterism and the development of larger scale, organizational forms of processing and dealing.

For the 1980s, Watson (ibid.) described the unusual non-profit orientation and cooperative productive arrangements operative in Warsaw, where commercialization of the Polish market was most evident. "Although most users produce drugs, they do so on an intermittent basis [and] all users [therefore] buy on the market from time to time. To produce drugs, typically three users form a temporary alliance. One will have access to poppy straw, another will provide a suitably safe flat for converting it to drugs and the third will sell the proportion designated for the market. After the costs of production have been covered, the profits are split." New users may begin by buying on the market but will soon be drawn to establishing a similar processing arrangement with others on the basis that it is cheaper and relatively easy. What has, in the past at least, been significant and unusual about the supply process in Poland is that, according to Watson (1991:13)

at no point does the accumulation of profit have any rôle to play. The farmers sell poppy straw on an opportunistic basis, either in exchange for goods unavailable in the villages, such as lightbulbs or tractor batteries, or to cover extra costs such as a daughter's wedding; drug users produce and sell to support their own drug use and as a means of subsistence" [emphasis in original].

95

Watson observes that

> there are similarities here with the lowest user-dealer levels
> of drug distribution in Britain . . . the crucial difference is
> that there is no commercial superstructure of producers or
> traffickers in it purely for the money. The result is that there
> is no tendency to expand the market, so the extent to which
> levels of consumption are supply driven is reduced.

For various reasons, including the convertibility of currency,
openness to western culture and ideas, identification as a prime
eastern European country ready for investment, etc., it is likely that
the Polish drugs market will in future become more westernized,
commercialized and criminalized: the intrusion of external market
forces will change the internal demand and supply structure and
Poland's recent drug market stability will go the way of the rest of
"the old system". In 1990, Chrusciel (1990: 12) observed that
"there are already records of cases of drug production destined for
illicit traffic; transit of drugs from Asia to Europe is increasing and
production for trafficking of amphetamine is growing" (see also
Boseley 1993).

Russia

Lee (1992: 184) has observed of the old Soviet Union that it was a
"country virtually self-sufficient in narcotics". Imports of heroin
and cocaine from the west showed evidence of increasing in the
early 1990s but remained a negligible part of the overall market.
However, officials are aware this could change as the Russian
economy becomes more integrated with the west (ibid.).

In 1992, United Nations officials investigating production of illicit drugs in seven of the former Soviet republics found that "From
Yalta to Alma Ata in Khazakstan" poppies, cannabis and drug
processing laboratories were commonplace. According to Boseley
(1993),

> in Khazakstan, even children ingest cannabis with sugar or
> milk. A single valley planted with 138,000 hectares of can-
> nabis can produce 5000 tonnes of marijuana. Cannabis

and opium are cultivated in Tadjikistan, which is also a through route to Moscow and the Baltic for Afghan opium and drugs are a common means of barter. The UN mission found opium poppies and cannabis in more than 3000 fields in Uzbekistan, crops certain to be more widely grown because more profitable than other cash crops. They reported that in 1991 a hectare of fruit earned between 15,000 (£15) and 20,000 roubles, a hectare of cotton 40,000 to 50,000 and a hectare of opium 2.5 million roubles. Even in Russia, where controls are tighter, synthetic drugs are being manufactured for export. The trade is going to be hard to stop with drugs costing about a tenth of their price in western Europe.

Synthetic drug production, mainly of amphetamines, but also the refining of morphine and heroin, has been discovered in Leningrad, Moscow, Riga, Perm, Rostov, Tomsk, Vladivostock and elsewhere (Lee 1992: 185–6). This suggests an extensive and well developed market yet Lee's research suggests that in the late 1980s the Russian drug market was still relatively low key, disorganized and non-commercial:

> users often acquire their supplies of narcotics from friends, associates or relatives. Some users obtain medicinal drugs (especially opiates such as morphine and codeine) through contacts in pharmacies, hospitals and medical storehouses. Money does not necessarily change hands in a drug transaction – if it does, the user may pay only a nominal sum (a fraction of the black market price) for a particular illicit substance. (Lee 1992: 186–7).

In the past, it seems that distribution has occurred through both friendship networks and more commercial market dealers. In the 1990s, as the Russian economy opens further to western influence and as organized criminal groups thrive (Bohlen 1993, Clark 1993) it is highly likely that the dynamics of the market will produce a fragmented and competitive but expansive and organized commerce in illegal drugs.

Summary

Overall, this latter description of the future for the Russian market, serves well as a description of European markets – east and west – more broadly. The tendency in the 1980s was towards small, fragmented, entrepreneurially active and adaptive, flexible but organized operations. For the successful drugs business, the notion that "small is beautiful" has its appeal (Dorn & South 1990; Dorn et al. 1992b). This tendency seems to remain dominant in the 1990s and is a conclusion with implications for control measures. Not least among these, is the importance of discarding popular and politically appealing notions that drug markets could be broken and destroyed "if only" enforcement operations could "get Mr Big", "smash the Mafia" or "track down the drug barons". As we have suggested, neither Italian nor British, or other European markets, are organized monopolies, or grand pyramids with clearly discernible tiers, or controlled by mafia cartels (see also Dorn 1993b).

Control measures: legal regulation and international controls in Europe

We are not primarily concerned in this book with issues to do with control, enforcement, regulation and law regarding drugs. However, as our discussion of the international dimensions of drug use and trafficking should suggest, and as will be apparent in our case studies, it is impossible to wholly separate the nature of drug markets from their interaction with law enforcement and control measures. Hence, in the final section to this chapter, we shall briefly sketch some pertinent history and current issues that deserve consideration alongside our central concerns. We shall conclude by considering the argument that enforcement responses are inherently flawed and counterproductive: the alternative path, according to these critics, is decriminalization or legalization of drug use. (Although the literature is sparse, for more detailed and specialized discussions of enforcement and legislation concerning drugs in Europe see: Dorn 1993c, 1994, Savona et al. 1994, Leroy 1991, Chatterjee 1989, Anderson 1989, Ch. 5, Hebenton & Thomas 1992, Albrecht & van Kalmthout 1989a, on decriminalization and legalization – for and against – see: Nadelman 1993, 1989, 1988, Trebach 1982, Wisotsky 1986, Inciardi 1991, Inciardi & McBride 1989, Courtwright 1993, Wilson 1990, South 1993, 1995a).

History

With the Shanghai Commission of 1909, the momentum of international meetings and agreements concerning the goal of drug control began its unsteady but eventually unremitting progress through the 20th century (Bruun et al. 1975, Albrecht & van Kalmthout 1989). European commitment to such efforts has always been seen as crucial, although enthusiasm has not always been as high as American prohibitionists hoped (De Kort & Korf 1992: 127–8).

In the late 19th century, perceptions of opium smoking and of international commerce in the drug underwent a change. Broadly speaking, opinion shifted from tolerance of medicinal and recreational use, and complicity in or acceptance of the trade, to growth of concern and agitation for some control over use and campaigning for cessation of the trade. The discussions of the Shanghai Commission (a fact-finding rather than decision making meeting) were followed by a conference with powers to draft an international treaty, brought together (despite some disinterest shown by Germany, Britain and the Netherlands) at the Hague in 1912 (Kort & Korf 1992: 127–8).

The interruption of the First World War meant that the drafted agreements concerning supervision and regulation of international trade and commitments to introduce domestic controls, were only ratified when peace came and they were incorporated into provisions of the Versailles Treaty, Article 295 (Bruun et al. 1975: 12). Through these agreements and subsequent pressures and reminders, the USA sought to re-emphasize its prohibitionist agenda – now fully articulated at home in the disastrous Great Experiment of alcohol prohibition. While a commitment of this nature was never likely to find much support from many of its wine-producing and alcohol-consuming League of Nations partners in Europe, nonetheless agreement about controls over other drugs, to work for the "gradual suppression of the abuse of opium, morphine and cocaine" (Bean 1974: 21), was less problematic. In part this was so because most European countries simply did not have much of a drug problem to suppress. In Britain for example, while official and popular concerns about use of these drugs had grown between the 1900s and 1920s, both concern and use were largely dissipated by the end of the 1920s (Berridge 1979, Pearson 1991, South 1994, Parssinen 1983). In such a context, all of the significant drugs legislation passed in Britain between 1920 and 1964 was, as Bean (1974: 35) notes, a matter of meeting the obligations of *international* treaties not a necessary response to some domestic drug problem.

In the era following the First World War, with the challenges of rebuilding economies and national morale, and of adjusting to a world now changed forever, it was unsurprising to find some public unease about media orchestrated images of the sinful and corrupting nature of drug use (e.g. Kohn 1992). Among governments and other authorities in Europe, the aim of suppressing drug use clearly had its supporters – but it also had opponents, as well as facing straightforward laxity in the implementation of the new restrictions (De Kort & Korf 1992: 128–30). In recent decades, most European countries have become signatories to and ratified major international agreements, most importantly the 1961 Single Convention on Narcotic Drugs (amended 1972), the 1971 Convention on Psychotropic Substances and the 1988 Convention (although many countries may have signed but not yet ratified the latter, see Leroy 1991). These treaties lay out schedules designating certain drugs to certain control categories based upon official perceptions of their danger to individuals and society, their legitimate medical value etc. More recently, international treaties and especially regional agreements within Europe have placed emphasis upon issues of mutual assistance concerning enforcement level co-operation, intelligence sharing, extradition, anti-money laundering strategies and so on (Dorn 1993 a,b, McLaughlin 1992: 480).

However, we should note that these varied international treaties and agreements can only lay out a *framework* for control-regulations in individual countries – they cannot dictate how provisions of the treaties will be interpreted or the extent to which they will be complied with. Hence a different picture may apply in different countries across Europe. Indeed, as a recent comparison of drug legislation in the countries of the European Community concluded:

Comparison of the legislation . . . reveals how far attitudes to the phenomenon and ways of controlling it vary. Differences in the way the role of the law is perceived reflect the different situation in each country and the lack of consultation between Member States in drawing up anti-drugs legislation. The only link of any kind holding them together in this respect was the fact that they had all ratified the 1961 United Nations Convention (Leroy 1991: 2).

Cross-border enforcement

Globally there are a number of regulatory and control agencies concerned with the international drug trade: several under the umbrella of the United Nations, plus other non-governmental organizations (Hartnoll, 1989: 38–9), as well as agencies aiming to foster co-operation between enforcement services such as the Customs Cooperation Council and Interpol (ibid.; Anderson 1989). Specifically in Europe, the number of agencies involved with responses to drug issues has risen with the profile of the subject. The Council of Europe Pompidou Group has been concerned with studies of drug issues, the European Community pursues interests in drug issues through three Directorates, and the European Parliament has initiated inquiries into drug problems and trafficking across member states (Hartnoll 1989: 39, Stewart-Clark 1986, Cooney 1991).

For our purposes here, Hopkinson (1991: 17–18) provides a useful summary of the politics and policy of European Community initiatives responding to international drug problems:

Many European groups deal with inter-governmental aspects of the drugs problem: the European Committee to Combat Drugs (CELAD) is the EC body responsible for co-ordinating member state anti-trafficking programmes and work undertaken in EC fora; the Trevi group organizes confidential meetings among government ministers (and others) to fight drugs and terrorism; the Schengen group comprises eight EC signatories who cooperate on policing following the abolition of internal border controls, and the

Pompidou group brings together 25 Council of Europe member countries and is encouraging closer co-operation with East Central Europe . . .

EC drugs policy co-operation started only in 1989 when the EC created CELAD as a ministerial level co-ordinating body. The European Programme for the Fight Against Drugs established five action areas in 1990: coordination of member states anti-drug policies, measures to stop drug trafficking, demand reduction, EC multilateral participation, and the creation of a European Observatory on Drugs (EOD) to monitor drug production, legislation, trafficking and demand.

The EC is considering anti-trafficking proposals including: more extensive checking at the EC external frontiers, including coast-lines; a common system of training and enforcement; harmonisation of anti-trafficking laws; a common visa policy for residents from third countries and immigrants; ground rules for "hot pursuit" of criminals from one country into another; spot checks of suspicious movements at borders; national drugs intelligence units to coordinate the work of police and customs officials; and an upgraded and common computerised system enabling the retrieval of information about international criminal profiles, trafficker types and methods of transport within seconds. At the July 1990 EC summit, it was agreed that a central European anti-drug agency or Europol would be created and that an EC system of control on precursor chemicals would be established.

It seems widely accepted that many moves towards international co-operation and exchange have been productive and beneficial. For example, Samson (1990: 41) observes that "the attachment of foreign police liaison officers to the Netherlands provides essential support to the enforcement efforts at the national level. Bilateral functional relationships with the enforcement authorities of Germany, the Scandinavian countries, France and the other Benelux countries are fostered through co-operation groups composed of officers from the participating countries." This system is similar to that operating in the UK and elsewhere in western Europe, especially where co-operation and mutual aid agreements are being given increasingly higher profiles and where the development of Europol has received strong support. However it is precisely in anticipation of this latter development that some pause for cautious thinking might be advisable.

The question is, what are the items on the control agenda in the 1990s and towards 2000? What exactly is expected of Europol in relation to its first target – drug trafficking? And how is it expected to go about it? For all its internationally known public image, Interpol offers little *operational* guidance (Anderson 1989) and the influence of the American Drugs Enforcement Administration in Europe has been to seek to "Americanize" European enforcement approaches and methods, sometimes helpfully but perhaps equally often, inappropriately (Nadelman 1990).

National police intelligence systems (e.g. in Britain and Italy) have been established with a *de facto* remit of targeting "top trafficking" yet as Dorn (1993b) points out, this is not a strategy that engages with the reality of trafficking in these countries or Europe more broadly. Such systems do not, therefore, offer a useful model for future policy or operational development. Some uncertainty about direction and rôle seems likely for the new agency. It would seem then that the "rocky path to Europol" (Hebenton & Thomas 1992) is not going to be much smoother in the short-run – while in the longer term, it is likely that a Europol which does prove to be effective will then face a whole new range of issues which have less to do with "catching the traffickers" and more to do with accountability and the question of "who controls the controllers?" (ibid.; McLaughlin 1992).

The prospects for legalization, decriminalization and harm reduction

While one response to ineffective control efforts is to pour in more resources, step up "the war" and get tougher on drugs – an increasingly powerful argument is that such a reaction is tired, discredited and counterproductive. In the USA, prime mover in international control efforts and keenest proponent of the need to conduct a "war" against drugs, there may be some signs of changing priorities. President Clinton may cut some drug enforcement funds for budget reasons as much as a desire to support treatment responses – but if so, then this is at least a start down a constructive path. Liberal media in the US already question the value of past policy (Treaster 1992) and emphasize the need for more adequate medical care and education as alternatives to the "drug war".

In Europe, the way forward, it is argued, must be to reduce the harm associated with drug use and related problems (e.g. legal, social, economic harms; O'Hare et al. 1992). To some degree, this can be accomplished within the present balance of the criminal justice and health system frameworks that many western European countries currently adopt (Dorn & South 1994). However, other countries, notably the Netherlands, offer a model for decriminalization which some observers argue should be followed elsewhere. Less clearly, proposals for a more radical form of complete legalization of drug use have also been made, but there are no concrete examples of this and it is harder to envisage in practice.

Essentially, the decriminalization proposal argues for tolerance of use of some drugs: in the Netherlands example, the aim of this policy and practice is to separate the cannabis market from the market for more dangerous drugs which Dutch law views as associated with "unacceptable risks". Cannabis remains an illegal drug, hence international conventions remain in force, but possession of small amounts of up to 30 grammes is regarded as a petty offence for which arrest is most unusual. Serious penalties and enforcement efforts are directed against the market for other drugs. This is one model that antiprohibitionists argue is sensible and easy to follow. The more extreme alternative, complete legalization, has many potential benefits but advocates of these are usually met by equally persuasive arguments about the costs that would be incurred (see e.g. Nadelman 1988, 1989, 1993, Courtwright 1993, Inciardi 1991). In favour, are the propositions that legalization would remove the basis for criminal profit and hence criminal organization and trade in drugs, violence and gang warfare would be cut, drug related crime would fall, drug users could be attracted into health, treatment and other services (e.g. HIV testing) if they no longer feared prosecution, and so on. Availability might hold steady, fall – or even increase, but even if it did, drugs would be purer, regulated, safer and taxation levied would pay for advice and treatment services.

Opponents respond that to follow this path would be morally, legally, ethically, socially, economically and politically wrong. Consumption would inevitably rise and bring higher health costs to individuals, social costs to families and medical costs to the state. Intoxicant related crime, violence and accidents would rise and, for those seeking drugs or strengths not offered by the legal outlets, then an illegal market would arise anyway, with the familiar attendant crime related problems. Furthermore, this whole debate has generally been carried out from a western, euro-centric, viewpoint and neglects the impact that legalization and consequent commercialization of drugs would have on third world countries which produce plant drugs: multinational firms would be likely to run a legal drugs agribusiness in ways which severely disrupt traditional patterns of farming and survival, potentially leading to poverty on a large scale.

There are some signs that while the weight of mainstream public and political opinion will, for the foreseeable future, remain balanced against legalization, there may be grounds for suggesting that a degree of incremental decriminalization is occurring and that, from ever more diverse sources, there is support for the idea that prohibitions have failed and that some alternative is needed. In Britain, possession of cannabis, and in some areas, of other drugs (in small amounts) has effectively been decriminalized by police cautioning policies and referral schemes which refer drug users away from the criminal justice system and towards help and advice agencies (Dorn & South 1994, Dorn 1993b). On the other hand, of course, the penalties for involvement with Class A and B drugs in Britain are severe, and for trafficking in heroin can invite a life sentence as well as seizure of assets (Dorn et al. 1992b, Ch. 10). In recent years, campaigning organizations like Release and the Legalise Cannabis Campaign, plus professional bodies like Justice and some senior police and probation officers, have rekindled debate about relaxation of possession laws. However, it is unlikely to be in Britain that major moves towards liberalization occur.

In Italy, prospects may be different. Despite support for anti-trafficking and anti-crime measures, the legal status of the drug user has received more restrained attention and possession of drugs for personal use has not generally been an offence. Jurists in Italy have disputed the constitutional value of drugs legislation, in particular those provisions which coerce users into treatment as an alternative to custody (Pisapia 1991). In terms of support for decriminalization, Italy has been one of the countries most active in the international "Anti-Prohibitionist League on Drugs". The Italian branch of this organization, founded in the mid 1980s, is related to the Italian Radical Party, which gained support throughout the 1970s on issues such as abortion, divorce law reform etc. In the late 1980s, a group of Radical Party members stood in the elections to the European Parliament under the banner of the Anti-Prohibitionist League – one of them won a seat and now speaks on behalf of the League in Parliament. Two lobbies can be distinguished within the Italian anti-prohibitionist movement. One calls for a system of public distribution of drugs, supervised by doctors and health authorities, the other advocates retailing of drugs in a free market, although subject to controls similar to those regulating alcohol and food production and distribution. There are differences of opinion between the two positions but both agree that to only legalize soft drugs would be to isolate users of hard drugs in a way which would be particularly damaging to them, leaving them to bear the brunt of control measures and the stigma of drug "abuse".

It is hard to see what the future holds for Europe on this issue. The Minority Group recommendations of the Stewart-Clarke Report (1986), produced by the European Parliament, argued that the EC should fund a serious study of the viability of antiprohibition measures which would be linked to information campaigns about the dangers of drug use (Diez-Ripolles 1989b). Some commentators on the European scene are pessimistic about the prospects for even modest liberalization (Boutmans 1989, Scheerer 1989) while others argue that it is inevitable: "it is . . . to be expected, almost predictable, that the world will see a trend towards the liberalization of narcotics. This liberalization will lead to a substantial breakdown of criminal organizations" (Wiarda 1989: 37). For this author, this process is certain to occur, so the important question is how to manage the integration of drugs into society.

Perhaps the point is, whether greater liberalization, decriminalization or whatever, does occur or not, increased drug use and availability will continue to be serious issues for societies across Europe for the foreseeable future. Policy makers and control-enforcers must acknowledge this, as one senior British police officer has done in urging policy makers, police and public to be prepared to "think the unthinkable" and consider "licensed drug supply" (Grieve 1993). Other commentators, as far apart on the control spectrum as "abolitionist theorist" Nils Christie (1989) and Interpol Director, Raymond Kendall (1993), seem to share some common ground – both agreeing that decriminalization of drug use is desirable and that police, courts and customs would still have a rôle to play in regulating a legal drugs market. In the development of a shared European policy, compromise and realism will be necessary, but pragmatic responses aimed at harm reduction and sensible use of resources will be a good starting point (South 1993, Caballero 1989, O'Hare et al. 1992).

4

Trafficking and distribution in London: competition, racism and enterprise in criminal labour markets

During the 1980s, the availability of illegal drugs and the nature of illicit markets in Britain changed dramatically. Distribution systems were transformed: from being highly localized and poorly structured they could now be described as extensive, widespread and systematically organized (Stimson 1987). Importation also changed, increasingly involving groups with no previous interest in the drug trade: "From reports of major seizures it appears that importers include professional criminals who are involved in several importations, and also business people who may indulge in one-off importations" (Stimson 1987: 48). A phenomenally profitable venture, drugs importation may pose risks but evidently both illicit and licit entrepreneurs find these are overshadowed by the potential rewards.

The reasons for these changes are complex. In part they are to do with generational developments in white professional crime groups: the retirement of old hands and the rise of the young, and the ideological spirit of 1980s entrepreneurialism that provided the climate in which this was occurring. They are also partly attributable to the activities of new criminal groups which are ethnically or geographically associated with those countries that produce and export drugs (see De Kort & Korf 1992). However, criminology has frequently exhibited a certain wariness when questions of race and crime are raised and hence, criminological studies of drug markets in Britain have so far avoided any straightforward statements on this issue. When we compare this situation with the US literature, where race and ethnic identity are crucial variables in analyses of drug markets and patterns of use, this seems a remarkable omission (see e.g. Trimble et al. 1992).

In this chapter we will describe structures of trafficking and distribution in England, with particular attention to London. In doing so we will review existing literature and draw upon our own findings and observations. We will also consider the diversity of participants, including ethnic groups, that are engaged in aspects and examples of drug-crime enterprises. While this approach addresses the neglected issue of race, our coverage is deficient in another sense. We have gathered little original material that contributes to discussions about women and drug use or dealing. We shall discuss issues such as the exploited rôle of women within the trafficking chain, being employed as couriers and suffering high sentencing costs when apprehended, and we shall note comments from women respondents and the relevant literature. But generally, this study is guilty of reporting drug worlds as male preserves.

Ethnic enterprise and trafficking

Two crucial features are usually regarded as ideal and necessary pre-conditions for the efficiency of a trafficking network. The first is impermeability with regard to police enquiries, the second – surprising as it may seem – is honesty in transactions and compliance with verbal agreements. Tyler (1986: 249) writes: "There are a couple of institutions that measure up excellently to such requirements. One is the blood family, the other is the expatriate ethnic community. Both have done well out of drugs trading".

Taking up this point we should first note two things. First, the vilification, persecution and victimization of various ethnic groups for real or imagined associations with drugs has been a strong constant of drug control history, since at least the late 19th century (Helmer 1975, Kohn 1992). Secondly, we acknowledge that sociological debate suggests that there are problems in developing analyses based on "categories" of race and ethnicity. As Carter & Green (1995) argue, sociologists would no longer subscribe to varieties of "scientific racism" but "race thinking" persists in a version with a strong interactionist pedigree. However, it seems to us that skin colour, cultural styles, differences, Otherness, do have consequences and implications for people in a racist world. To begin to illuminate the way racism in the drug economy may operate and parallel racism in the legitimate economy, we must accept this.

Chronologically, it is the Chinese community that is generally cited as the first to have been involved in drug importation and distribution in England. Since the late 19th century, Chinese entrepreneurs are said to have carried out business within their own communities and without disturbance, drawing upon ancient customs of reciprocity and a system of payment based entirely on trust (Tyler 1986, Kohn 1992). A sophisticated system for laundering money has helped maintain this degree of invisibility and the scope of activity is impossible to evaluate. In the 1960s and 1970s, heroin bought in the Golden Triangle, and routed through Hong Kong, would reach London concealed among other items imported for the Chinese immigrant community. Underground banking would then guarantee the invisibility of profits. Within the Chinese community, one such underground system is known as "chop shop". A similar system is known by different names in different regions: "Amongst those from the Indian subcontinent it is known as 'chiti' banking, 'hundi' banking or 'hawalla' banking. And among some of the Latin American peoples it is known as 'stash-house banking'" (Nove 1991: 5). Such sub rosa systems consist of banking and other services provided by a branch, a partner or a relative of the immigrant group operating in their country of origin. The system provides mechanisms for the notional or actual transfer of money or credit between branches, for the conversion of funds from one currency to another, and for the repatriation of funds when required (South 1992; Nove 1991). Family ties ensure that the essential element of trust is maintained despite the potential problems that distance and secrecy might cause. "In many cases no single member of the family knows quite how many parts there are to the network, and secrecy is thus assured" (Nove 1991: 7).

The next ethnic group closely identified with heroin importation were Iranians, active in the early 1980s. As described in Chapter 2, heroin is alleged to have constituted a currency for middle-class migrants escaping from the new regime of the Ayatollah. Among this group, were to be found students who had used heroin while living in Iran and who "sidelined" in trafficking while continuing a student career in Britain.

The successors to Iranian importers are purported to be entrepreneurs from the Pakistani community, who have expanded their participation since around the mid 1980s when the Pakistani variety of heroin gained a virtual monopoly on the London market. These entrepreneurs work with partners who reside in the producer country and act as mediators with local growers. The areas where poppy is grown, such as the district of Dir, are inhabited by traditional tribes which are administered by means of informal institutions, or village councils also called jirga (di Gennaro 1991). According to Labrousse (1991) the rich families of Karachi are either the owners of the land where poppy grows or enter into close commercial partnerships with them. They buy the product, or sometimes commission it, and after the refining process, export it to countries where their branch-partners reside. The significance of this trafficking channel was recognized in the mid to late 1980s when Pakistan became the focus of international interventions, including United Nations' support for law enforcement "crackdowns" and crop substitution and rural development schemes. In Britain, anxiety and xenophobic concern went hand in hand and the Government increased contributions of financial and military aid to Pakistan to assist in its drug war efforts (ibid.).

Heroin coming from Burma is allegedly always shipped westward via India and some Indian-origin entrepreneurs based in Britain will be among those groups which act as end-destination importers. Commercial skills and the maintenance of familial and commercial relationships in India facilitate involvement in trafficking (Tyler 1986). Nigeria is regarded as one of the other key staging posts for heroin entering Britain (McCarthy & Kirby 1990). Particular surveillance and intelligence efforts are therefore directed at travellers and cargoes arriving from Nigeria, resulting in high annual seizures. Nigerian couriers or "mules" caught attempting to smuggle drugs now form the largest single group of foreign prisoners in British prisons (ILPS 1990). Research conducted by the Inner London Probation Service found that several Nigerians arrested for smuggling originally had no intention of carrying drugs. However, when seeking funds for their travel they had approached moneylenders, friends or relatives for loans and "were told they would be given a free return ticket, plus a sum of money, if they would agree to carry some drugs and deliver them to a certain address after leaving the airport. . . . In one case, a Nigerian female carrying drugs worth over £28,000 was given a plane ticket plus £400 and told to give back the change on the return to Nigeria" (ILPS 1990: 46). Research conducted by Green (1991) revealed that 72 per cent of persons imprisoned for illegal importation of drugs were foreign nationals. "Africans combined account for 35% of this population, with the largest national category being Nigerian (30% of the total)" (Green 1991: 5). In June 1990, 26 per cent of women under sentence were known to have been convicted of drugs offences, compared with 8 per cent of men. At the same time, 26 per cent of women in prison were of ethnic minority origin, compared with 17 per cent on 30 June 1985. This unprecedented increase is attributed to the growing number of drug related offences committed by women. "Many of the women are drug couriers from other countries, who will be deported after serving a prison sentence" (Nacro 1991: 2).

Traffickers may frequently attempt to conceal the source country or region from which imports originate and hence drugs are likely to pass through other countries not immediately identified as drug producing areas. According to HM Customs and Excise (1990), more than 40 per cent of drugs entering Britain come via other European Community countries. The Greek islands, the Dutch ports of Rotterdam and Amsterdam, and the southern coast of Italy are singled out as high risk locations from where drugs are imported to Britain (*The Guardian*, 11 October 1990).

Import operations and distribution are not likely to be conducted by the same groups. While the large majority of apprehended importers are foreign nationals, these importers generally do not have the means and contacts to enter into the distribution of drugs. They therefore sell the commodity on, to locally established figures who are in a better position to supply local markets. These may be seen as wholesale distributors who have direct contact with importers and with locally based middle-range distributors.

"Traditional villains": from armed robbery to drug distribution

Examples of importers and wholesale distributors are now reported to be common among traditional white villains who in past decades would have been more likely to be involved in "project crimes" such as armed robbery (McIntosh 1975). The shift towards drug-crime was encouraged by the belief that it yields high profits, easily made, while the increasing use of firearms in robberies was now being countered by the arming of police, making such ventures rather more dangerous. Investments in drug deals were deemed safer and armed robbery has largely been left to "nutters or cowboys . . . dangerous amateurs who impulsively rush in demanding money and firing guns in all directions" (Taylor 1984: 92).

An account of the dual-career of Roy Garner, a well known London criminal and for a time, less well known police informant, describes this shift:

> When the 1980s dawned, Roy Garner was as quick as every other gunman in town to see that the golden age of armed robbery had passed. New types of crime beckoned and the professionals moved effortlessly into massive tax frauds and drug dealing. The temptations were overwhelming. . . . There were big sentences for drug trafficking but the use of couriers made for relatively small risks. (Jennings et al. 1990: 105)

Other journalistic accounts echo Garner's story and confirm that, after initial resistance to drug dealing, many professional criminals "soon realized that here was a new way of making money that required no getaway car and ran less risk of informers. It had the added advantage that there was no victim running to the police" (Campbell 1990: 5).

Dorn et al. (1992b, Dorn & South 1990) describe such groups as "criminal diversifiers" and report their continued involvement in a range of traditional activities – such as theft and distribution of goods, and semi-legitimate businesses such as used-car dealerships. Such businesses may produce a legitimate profit but also provide a "front" for other activities. The autobiography of Charlie

Richardson, a notorious criminal of the 1960s, provides a good illustration: "I bought stolen metal and sold it to people who knew a lot of it was stolen. . . . Like any good entrepreneur I had to feel I was growing and diversifying all the time" (Richardson 1991: 104–6). Richardson exemplifies the wheeling and dealing culture which came to include drugs as just another commodity to be bought, sold and moved: "Each day of my life was filled with a variety of ideas and transactions. I revelled in my ability to switch from selling metals to buying shoe polish to opening a new company. With all my companies I enjoyed working out the transfer of assets and debts from one to the other. I juggled ideas, people, money, business and commodities all day." (ibid.: 130).

In areas such as North Southwark and Bermondsey, the legacy of the traditional criminal gangs of the 1950s and 1960s was passed to a new generation of illegal entrepreneurs who came into their own in the late 1970s and 1980s. Hobbs (1988: 117–18) describes a similar entrepreneurial culture in East London, where the peculiarities of the local economic structure "required generation upon generation of individuals to acquire and internalize the essential characteristics of the business entrepreneur. . . . The East End entrepreneur deals and trades in commodities and services within the parameters of a localized version of legitimate business practice". Capital accumulated from traditional semi-legal trades may then be re-invested in enterprises such as drug importation or distribution.

All the above seem to indicate that in London wholesale or large-scale drug distribution is the preserve of indigenous groups formed by white English nationals. These groups have not only traditionally monopolized the distribution of other illegal goods, but are also prepared to discourage competition by any means available. Their intimate knowledge of the networks within which goods are exchanged puts them in a position to deal with middle-range distributors to whom they sell units of their imported drugs. Middle-range distributors are usually in contact with specific communities and with street dealers operating in those communities. At this level individuals and small groups are already involved in a variety of activities in the "irregular economy". This economy, which is multiracial in nature, is a crucial channel for the distribution of illicit drugs, as it provides a "facilitating" subculture, a previously acquired expertise, and a series of structures and rôles: "The irregular economy provides multiple conduits for the distribution and exchange of drugs, and for a variety of other goods and services, prostitution, the disposal of stolen goods, and so on" (Auld et al. 1986: 172). Within this economy, the pub, drinking club and pool-hall have been useful and important distribution outlets, where middle-range drug traders have sold to retail dealers (Power 1987).

Race, racism and drug markets

We can now return to the little-discussed issue of race, racism and the drug economy. The majority of ordinary couriers detected and receiving a prison sentence are African, Afro-Caribbean and Latin Americans, with a high proportion being women. Whether this reflects a bias in the intelligence profiling that informs customs surveillance, is open to debate. However, leaving aside the possibility of institutionalized racism, it is likely that the high number of foreign travellers from poor, drug producing areas, who are involved in importation into Britain, is due to the fact that these are the individuals most easily coaxed, bribed or tricked into acting as "mules". The riskiest and most stigmatized tasks in domestic and international aspects of the drug economy are left to unskilled criminal labourers who are often poorly paid (Ruggiero 1994). These, with some exceptions, are non-British nationals whose rôles are limited to smuggling and then passing on the drugs imported. Large scale importers, of whatever background, are not usually directly involved in the smuggling itself – they organize transit between point of departure and arrival. Thereafter they are likely to "sell-on", employing pre-established commercial relationships with (usually) white distributors, who already provide other illegal goods and services in their localities. One middle-range dealer described examples of such local distributors:

These are people who deal quantities around 100 grammes and are very well known in the community. They sell to a number of street dealers whom they trust. Some of these distributors do not make a real career in crime, in the sense that they don't increase each time the quantity of drugs they deal with. They don't monopolise the market nor do they eventually become international traffickers. They'd rather open up a clean business or just boost their previous business. Often they continue to sell drugs on the side even when they become more respectable. In this way they still maintain a high status in the community both as entrepreneurs and as tough lads, as they were in the past.

If they can, it makes sense for established "traditional" crime groups (principally white) to keep at some distance from the level of international trafficking and importation. To do so can increase security and profit. They can hold – or at least attempt to exert – a virtual monopoly of control over their local markets and are therefore in a position of some strength when negotiating terms with importers. Importers may hold a commodity for which there is a large demand – but offloading it in small, saleable units is not an easy matter. In terms of added value, this segment of the distribution chain can be more financially rewarding than other segments of the drug economy. Interviews conducted in Brixton confirm this argument and draw attention to the development of a distinctive racial division of labour in parts of the London drug economy. One interviewee, a black street dealer, described examples of this division:

> There are about 12 middle-range distributors who never go out on the street in this area. They take between 50% and 70% of the street value of the drugs sold. In turn, they buy in other areas. It is very rare that distributors here are in direct contact with importers, or are importers themselves. Those who buy from importers live in more white respectable areas and are usually white British.

Dealers operating in Brixton explicitly argued that even the so-called Yardies find it hard to gain control of any of the more remunerative segments of the drug economy. One respondent argued that white professional criminals, not the police, have ensured that the Yardies have been unable to build up significant and sizeable criminal businesses. He also suspected that white criminal groups undermined the potential danger of competition by keeping the police informed of anything incriminating, or of possible immigration offences. In this way, the police intelligence system has acquired information "about the Yardies that they would never have picked up by themselves" (Ruggiero 1993a). This is not, of course, by any means a new phenomenon. Rivals in drug distribution and crime generally, have always been good potential sources of information for the police (Pritchard & Laxton 1978: 47, Dorn et al. 1992b: 130–1). After the tragic killing of PC Patrick Dunne in Clapham in October 1993, the popular press seized on images of black "Yardie" gangsters with automatic weapons fighting for a share in the crack-cocaine trade. Such images are potent and doubtless symbolic. In reality "there is no Yardie mafia. The relatively small number of violent criminals – 30 or 40 – who have come to Britain from Jamaica have little by way of organization. . . . Put simply, the so-called Yardies are illegal immigrants. They bring drugs and expertise on crack dealing and expect to make large profits" (Nelson & Victor 1993). However, there are limits to the success and scope of such activity and there are few signs here of the development of truly "organized" crime (ibid.; Porter & Elliott 1993).

Prejudice and stereotyping are as common in the drug economy as the legal economy, consequently black dealers find it extremely hard to climb the distribution hierarchy. Those who do succeed may be viewed by white participants in the drug business with some suspicion, not so much for being drug dealers as for being entrepreneurs: moral disapproval of relatively prosperous black drug distributors simply reflects common prejudice against the black population, rather than against drug dealers. A dealer operating in Brixton affirmed that even in the crack business, allegedly controlled by black entrepreneurs, the position of blacks is in fact confined to the lower strata of the distribution chain. They would buy cocaine from white, large-scale suppliers, and then "wash" it before selling on the street. "The good stuff", he said, "is kept outside of Lambeth". Mixed support for this account can be found in the recent research by Bean & Pearson (1992) on crack distribution in Nottingham. There they found that:

> Many of the subjects claimed to know about the major crack suppliers but made contradictory statements which no doubt reflected the secrecy that surrounded them. Some said most suppliers and dealers were Afro-Caribbean

while others thought that the major suppliers were white American and London business men *"who get the black guys to do all the work"* (ibid.: 27; emphasis added).

In terms of the accounts from street dealers in Lambeth, the reports from Bean & Pearson are not that contradictory at all: small to medium scale black dealers are known to operate in the drug economy of south London, their contention is that larger scale distributors and suppliers are predominantly white.

Such observations are not, of course, new or unique. Lindesmith's (1965) classic work indicated the exclusion of blacks from managerial positions in the drugs economy of various cities in the northern USA. Redlinger (1975) provides a similar analysis in his detailed case study of the heroin market in San Antonio, Texas and the competing involvements of blacks, Mexicans and whites. Redlinger argues that whites can have access to and do well in legitimate occupations, therefore any failure in the heroin market is not crucial to them. However, noting the argument that minorities have traditionally used illegal occupations as routes to upward mobility, Redlinger (1975: 351) observes that in Texas, the illicit heroin market may offer such a route to Mexican-Americans but not to blacks.

> Blacks are not only denied access to legitimate occupations, but in addition, to illegitimate ones as well. . . . This situation is not unique to San Antonio or to the illicit heroin market. . . . [For example] Blacks who at one time controlled the rackets in their areas have lost control to whites and have been relegated to the lowest positions in the hierarchy (e.g. Cloward & Ohlin 1961: 199–202).

We suggest that the structure of the drug economy mirrors characteristics of the legal economy. In other words, wider social disadvantage based on race is reflected in the disadvantaged positions occupied by non-white citizens in the drug business. Traditional white groups frequently occupy the segments of the drug business where safer operations are conducted and more profit is generated. Blacks, other minorities, the "foreigners" – are blocked in their careers, be they legal or illegal.

The London drug market: patterns and participants

The spread of drug use in Britain, in particular heroin, seems to have been facilitated by a number of factors. Interestingly, when we think of London in a comparative context, it appears that some of these factors may be "peculiarities of the English" and their drug markets. As already suggested, one key factor was that many of the drugs which have become widely used since the 1970s could be smoked or sniffed and snorted – cannabis, of course, but also heroin, amphetamine, cocaine and later, crack-cocaine – thus overcoming cultural taboos against injecting. Another facilitating circumstance was the relative purity of drugs available in British cities such as London. Research conducted in Spain, France and Italy, for example, indicated that unreliable levels of purity and the unknown percentage of additives in street drugs, were one important barrier to drug experimentation (Funes & Romani 1985, Aspe 1992, Ruggiero 1992). Continental European neophytes may, therefore, have been attracted to drug use but, at least for a while, held back because of reputedly low or unpredictable purity. It is the relatively high purity of drugs in the British market that seems to be what keeps attracting users from abroad. Many Italian heroin users, for example, choose to settle in London less for its tourist attractions or the services and support offered by drug agencies, than because of its reputation for relatively high purity levels (Dianin, Duckworth & Lipsedge 1991).

There is another important difference between London and other European cities: in Rome, Paris, Madrid and elsewhere, administrative and police rules require that everybody officially registers precisely where they live. Residence certification, obligatory in many European contexts, is unheard of in British cities where people can literally get lost. Hence, when compared to other European cities, residential mobility and absence of registration may facilitate drug distribution in London. As one ex-user recollects:

> The dealer I bought from for about two years moved at least five times. He came from East London, and then moved south of the river, where initially nobody knew him. Every three or four months, when I went to score, he would tell me that the next time he would be at another address.

His customers remained the same, and it was on us to follow him around to his new addresses.

High mobility does not arouse suspicion in London, where many residents – especially the young, transient students and tourists – seem to pursue a lifestyle of permanent nomadism. This is not to argue that enforcement effectiveness would be enhanced by the introduction of residency notification or identity cards (also common in the rest of Europe). There may be arguments to support this view and some police officers have suggested ID cards would be helpful, but there are also serious concerns that are raised by such a prospect. In the context of the free movement of individuals across European borders, recent Government proposals to introduce identity cards for welfare claimants, the introduction of machine-readable passports and so on, these issues are likely to receive further debate in the 1990s.

Another factor which may have contributed to the spread of serious drug use in Britain can be found in the way retail distribution is actually conducted in most of its urban areas. Descriptions of "street" dealers and "street" cultures convey a certain image of drug use and markets. However in reality, much (possibly most) drug dealing transactions in London and England actually take place behind closed doors – off the street, on private premises, within private homes. This is the case in both metropolitan and rural areas (Bolton & Walling 1993). Arguably this exposes British users to less risk of attracting police attention than their continental European counterparts. "Street dealing" may be more of a routine reality in other European cities and when applied to London should be qualified by recognition of the wide range of other, less public, venues in which dealing takes place. To note just two obvious examples, which seem to have been paid surprisingly little attention in ethnographies of drug dealing in Britain, ideal private–public spaces for drug distribution include the pub and the nightclub. For example, in the Notting Hill and Bayswater areas of west London, several pubs are well known for drug dealing – and several more are less well known. Popular perception of drug problems and drug dealing in this area probably focuses on the market for cannabis around All Saints Road (Dorn et al. 1992b: 103–11). However, the wider area is also a centre for tourism, the music industry, publishers, antique dealers, meeting places like restaurants and cafes; and it is extremely cosmopolitan with residents and visitors from the east, Middle East, Africa, Australasia, Europe and North and South America. In short, there is demand for a variety of drugs from a variety of consumers, the area is well placed to be a centre for drug importation, outward distribution and overspill into local markets, and numerous pubs and clubs facilitate this. One pleasantly decorated pub, fairly centrally placed on the tourist track, managed for years to combine a healthy legitimate trade as an outwardly respectable pub while hosting dealers in heroin, cocaine and amphetamine, high class prostitution and pornographic videos. The use of nightclubs in distribution has been described by Dorn et al. (1992b) in two case studies: "Ari" and "Leo" used Leo's south coast nightclub "as a contact and sales point [from which] they started to sell lots of 100 grammes to established dealers on a cash-up-front basis. When in full operation – which lasted about two years – the organization was moving up to one kilo of heroin per week" through the nightclub and another site (ibid.: 57). On a smaller scale, the case study of "Abby" also describes distribution of a drug (MDMA – ecstasy) through the club scene of London and south coast towns and, in this case, the relationship between dealing, music and style, rather than dealing and profit (ibid.: 6–10). Some mix of the two can be found in Elliott's (1992) account of semi-organized and tolerated in-house dealing in a central London dance club in the early 1990s. Elliott had worked as a member of the security staff and made field-work notes on his observations of the social organization of the club and, in particular, the different participants in drug distribution in and around the club. To provide a structure for his observations he adopted the typology proposed by Dorn & South (1990). Elliott describes corruption within the club security team, headed by "Steve" who he classes as a small-scale "criminal diversifier". It was not clear to what extent the club management colluded with, simply tolerated or were ignorant of the drug dealing in the club – though complete ignorance of such activity seems unlikely. Here Elliott describes the different dealer rôles that could be identified:

> Rather than working on the front door, Steve travelled through the club as a benefactor to the punters. While his

security team enforced their authority, Steve made sure that his dealers were stocked for the evening ahead. Many of these dealers were usually inside the club before the club was open for legitimate business. This included DJ's who had their own market among their fans. So the dealers themselves fell into three main groups:

1. "House Dealers", who generally worked for Steve;
2. "Night Dealers", who were known to house dealers and worked on a commission basis either inside the club or more normally away from the club in their own home areas (e.g. scoring at the club and taking the drugs back to their locality, perhaps out of town, for re-sale; see the case of Abby, the ecstasy dealer noted above for a similar example).
3. Persons who mixed characteristics of the "Mutual Society" and the "Trading Charity" categories, who, on the whole, bought their drugs from one of the above to distribute to their friends that night. This group were the principal consumers in the market and hence were the largest group. . . . [However, as Elliott observes] it is reasonably clear that some of these groups were intertwined (e.g. Steve, the "criminal diversifier" was also sidelining from a legitimate business).

Firearms and violence in drug markets

It may be that in the 1990s, drug markets, particularly those for cocaine and crack, will become more volatile, prone to risk-taking, and likely to make further moves into street areas that distributors attempt to control, a process which may also involve increased use of firearms. We should note, however, that the relationships between firearms, drug dealing and profitability, are not as straightforward as frequently portrayed. Commonly, use of firearms is explained as the outcome of turf wars fought for the control of areas producing high profits; or in terms of the combination of high profitability and heavier sentences for drug-crime making the cost-benefit calculation one which favours use of firearms against rivals or enforcement officers. However, in some cases, the increasing use of firearms may suggest that the stakes being played for are getting lower, not higher. In parts of south London it is not the successful entrepreneurs who carry guns to impress and occasionally use them to settle disputes, it is the small dealers on the street, the ones with no future and no other way of making an impact. At the same time, the broader context is one where increasing competition both increases the potential for conflict and readiness to use firearms while it pushes down profits. Hence, the highly visible, open, street dealing markets most associated with use of firearms and violence, may generate considerable amounts of money overall – but, the individual or group working in such markets will be making relatively lower profits than in less competitive market places.

In London, parts of the Kings Cross area may fit this argument (Miles 1992), as well as areas of South London and Moss Side, Manchester (Dorn et al. 1992b: 37–41). Bean & Pearson (1992) report similar trends in their case study of one area of Nottingham describing changes in crack and cocaine use between 1989–90 and 1991–92. In 1989–90 various dealers operated from "off-street" sites such as private houses, pubs and clubs but by 1991–92, two major changes had occurred in terms of availability. "Firstly, crack was readily available while cocaine powder was not, and secondly, far from the need to make the secretive contacts with dealers described in 1989/90, crack was offered for sale and could be bought 24 hours a day on the street and in the clubs in the area" (Bean & Pearson 1992: 26–7).

This study also reports increased use or threat of use of firearms. Note also the exploitative division of labour whereby distributors employ others as their enforcers: "In 1991/92 the police were aware of the increased presence of firearms on the crack scene and certainly the researcher met dealers who said they owned guns. She was told that the collection of crack debts was enforced by illegal immigrants from Jamaica sponsored by local suppliers."

Participants and characteristics

In the London drug market of today, the differentiation of "social types" involved in drug use seems much wider than two decades ago and respondents (black and white) were almost unanimous in arguing that to talk of "drug use" *per se* is problematic. Patterns, styles and effects of use differ depending on a range of variables: people use different mixtures of drugs, effects differ according to strength and composition, the conditions in which drugs are administered, the expectations of users, their activities, their social rôle, their self-perception, and the labels applied to them (Becker 1963, 1967). Bearing all this in mind, we will now examine some relevant studies which identify characteristic social features of drug users in Britain, and at the same time we will compare these with our own findings.

Although drug use is spread widely across social groups in modern Britain, we concentrate here on the most visible sector of users, those who are most vulnerable and most stigmatized. These are the individuals and groups tied into localized drug and criminal networks or those whose main problem is that they have no ties at all, who drift into and out of social encounters and geographical areas. Many of these will have regular or periodic involvement in the semi-legal economy, and/or straightforwardly criminal economy. Examples of the former are found both in industrial life and in the tertiary sector, where underpaid, precarious and "invisible" (no tax, no national insurance, non-unionised etc.) jobs are offered and perks, fiddles and other hidden reward systems are common (Mars 1982, Scraton & South 1984). In the latter, we find the circulation and exchange of illegal commodities such as stolen goods and drugs (Sutton 1993, Foster 1990, Auld et al. 1986). In recent economic conditions of stagnation, inflation, high unemployment, the forcing down of wage levels and the expansion of the tertiary sector, the conditions have been right for a degree of blurring across the boundaries between these two economies.

Hence it may be quite common for some of those employed in informal labour markets to make intermittent forays in both directions. While active in the unpredictable, hidden market for labour and goods which, to borrow the term that Henry (1978) nicely employs, we might refer to as an arena of "borderline crime" – some individuals may, at the same time, engage in activities which have clearly gone over the edge of the borderline and into the criminal economy. Such individuals (defined by Gallo & Ruggiero (1985) as "delinquent-workers"), may sooner or later encounter illicit drugs and in time, turn to use and dealing. As Auld et al. (1986: 173) argue "people get involved in aspects of the irregular economy, and it is through their involvement in this partially petty-criminal economy that they may come to buy, exchange, sell and consume heroin". This kind of labour market analysis is perhaps more useful than simplified accounts of causal links between unemployment and drug use.

However, not everyone encounters the market in the same way or at the same level – neither drug users/dealers nor "the market" are homogeneous, undifferentiated categories. Buying, exchanging, selling and consuming drugs are not always, and automatically, meshed together. In part, this is because *laissez faire* principles do not prevent the emergence of hierarchies: to the contrary, the value and profit potential related to drugs as commodities stimulate a division of labour in the market that implies tighter organization, principles of reliability and credit, and other devices which mirror the demands of legal enterprises (cf. Johnson et al. 1990). In one illustrative account from a South London dealer:

> People tend to think that it is very easy to get hold of a quantity of stuff and go around selling it. In fact, you must know the right people and be known by them as reliable. You can be using the stuff, all right, but you also have to show that you keep in control and are respected in the scene. You must know your way around and always be on the ball. If you follow the rules you get enough stuff for yourself plus some to sell. Also, if you are all right you get good stuff, otherwise you only get lousy quality.

Many young people (white and black) that were interviewed did not see formal work (especially the type of work they could reasonably aspire to) as an enduring source of status and identity. Hence, simplistic responses to the "unemployment causes drug use/dealing" proposition may be regarded as patronizing and unrealistic if they can only offer "alternatives" of low level "dead-end" work. The rights and wrongs of such perceptions are debatable but such a debate should emphasize that what is at issue is not simply the problem of unemployment but the *quality* of jobs and life on offer. For such young people, the less structured informal economy and adjacent illegal economy do seem to have attractions. However, whether this attractiveness persists for those whose involvement in the drug economy comes to dominate their lives, is open to doubt.

De-skilled and routine labour in drug markets: the coming of the "mass" criminal?

We use the term "mass" criminal here to convey the idea of drug related petty-criminality as a form of "de-skilled" labour, performed by the "street-wise" but in circumstances that constrain them and which they will rarely break out of. Such contributors to the drug economy are found across the globe: they ensure the success and reproduction of drug markets despite all enforcement efforts and triumphs. They are interchangeable, replaceable, powerless, moveable, dependent. The work of "mass" criminals implies a routinization of tasks, a specific set of rôles, a fixed place in the division of labour and a virtually stagnant career (in terms of related, broader sociological debates see the growing literature on Fordism/Post-Fordism, e.g. Jessop et al. 1991). Follow-up studies of drug user/dealer careers do indeed show how their activities and lifestyle may occasionally involve enterprise, energy and even a frenetic pace, but these do not produce upward social mobility. The "Taking care of business" perspective on the active life of the drug user is an important counter to stereotypes of the dazed, dozing and incapable junkie. However, such activity is still likely to involve dull routines of scoring, using, seeking funds, involvement in dealing, petty crime, avoiding the police, failing to avoid them and facing the criminal justice system, social workers, probation, prison and so on.

One description of the routine work of users was provided by researchers investigating the drug scene in Earls Court. Here a hierarchy of dealers was found whereby lower level sellers would only be allowed to handle one or two £20 wraps. These "workers" were subjected to strict discipline by means of threats and violence from their "employers". Despite all this, their work was not "secure", but occasional, thus encouraging users into a never-ending search for new (but similar) earning activities. Their provision of drugs, in other words, was never guaranteed. The researchers report: "Such sub-contracted work was often short-term and irregular, as was the case when three users were hired to sell thirty-four ounces of heroin that had come into the Earls Court area" (Jones & Power 1990: 15).

Routine occupational hazards include encounters with the criminal justice and treatment systems. Wiepert et al. (1977) found that almost all the heroin users followed-up in their career had received a court conviction for repeated, similar offences. Gordon (1983) found that criminality rather than addiction was the key characteristic of a sample of 60 drug clinic patients followed up after 10 years:

> The extensive and continued criminality of these patients remains their main characteristic. It is difficult to conceive of a patient group, presenting primarily for medical care, who could approach a conviction rate of 97%. The continuation of criminal behaviour at follow-up was predicted on arrival at the clinic by a record of conviction *before* drug abuse and poor educational attainment" (ibid.: 172; emphasis added).

For these habitual users, the experience of the "revolving door" of encounters with the criminal justice and treatment systems had not enabled them to improve their skills and move out of a drug lifestyle and the drug economy. The fact that most of them had also employed violence while repeating the same offences over the years seems to underline the increasingly tough and competitive nature of the drug scene. Jarvis & Parker's (1989) study of 46 London-based heroin users showed that their annual rate of conviction more than doubled following the onset of regular heroin use. Such users might be involved in transferring considerable wealth, in the form of drugs, cash or stolen goods, from one place to another and from one person to another, but their personal profit is likely to be slim and primarily consist of payment in small amounts of drugs. Moreover, "Despite the glamour of the setting and the considerable sums of money involved, many subjects described repetitive lifestyles of dull uniformity" (ibid.: 182).

While many studies link increased drug use with increased criminality, the debate about "which comes first?" – delinquent and criminal associations or drug use – has produced a considerable literature (South 1994; 1995b). Certainly it seems over-simplistic and unsupported by evidence to suggest that there is a direct causal relationship between the two. In the case of the argument that drug use "causes" crime, it is interesting to note the findings of research conducted in Camden, Islington and Westminster which illustrates the point that drug using careers are not *necessarily* linked to criminal careers (O'Brian 1989). The development of a drug habit, with a consequent increase in the quantity of drug required, caused unsustainable financial difficulties for some, resolved by abstaining rather than trying to increase illicit earnings.

These studies may differ in their implications for the "causality" debate but confirm that profitable careers in the drug economy are not that easy to develop.

The growth of the drug economy and the decline of the "craft of crime"

Despite the emphasis placed by media and some enforcement sources, on the sensational aspects of drug related crime – most of it is, of course, fairly unsensational. In an area of criminality that is undoubtedly highly significant in terms of international growth, profit generation, scope for corruption and so on, it is important to emphasize that most drug related crime is petty, disorganized, opportunistic and very unsophisticated. The increase in the number of drug related offences and offenders does not herald, in Britain at least, a dramatic growth of "organized" crime. Rather, at the higher and middle levels of the market, criminal groups that are organized but not in a united manner, are found. A degree of business acumen and professionality characterizes their activities. At the lower levels, professionality, flair and "know-how" may still be seen as desirable by some but increasingly such qualities are unimportant to many others who are engaged in drug related crime. With a touch of irony, we might note recurrent arguments about declining standards and levels of skill generally in modern society and speculate on whether a decline in criminal skills exhibited by those involved in the drug economy reflects a general "decline in standards" in the "craft of crime" even while crime rates *per se* increase (McIntosh 1975, Hobbs 1993).

Recently, senior police officers have made statements linking rising crime levels to both recession and economic hardship (Loveday 1992: 19). Thus,

Disclosing an 11% rise in recorded crime in the Metropolis

129

for 1991, a police spokesman commented that the increase had to be viewed against a "backcloth of recession" and that the very high increase in street robberies [26%] was recorded in inner-city areas of London which had experienced "tough times in terms of their social and economic position" (*Independent* 19 February 1992) (Loveday 1992: 19–20).

Such interpretations invite debate about the complex relationships between unemployment and crime (Box 1987) and the significance of the drug economy (recently for example, Labour MP Frank Field gave a Justice in Society lecture in which he argued that "the drug economy is filling the void left by long-term unemployment", *The Observer*, 7 November 1993). Here we simply wish to draw attention to the fact that just as the formal labour market can be seen as stratified by skill levels, so too can the unemployed labour force *and the criminal labour market*. Thus, when considering general trends we might more specifically ask about the "quality" of the crimes being committed – meaning "quality" in terms of professionality, expertise, craft, planning versus opportunism etc. Is the investment of skill and professionality in crime declining?

The implication of all this is that much low-level drug-related crime is becoming increasingly unskilled and hazardous. Carrying out drug related property crime at a level which provides substantial financial reward is not easy or simple. Target hardening and the decline of criminal crafts and skills contribute to this. Low-level street-dealing is targeted by low-level law enforcement (Murji 1993). Small, disorganized, unprofessional dealers are picked up and lose out; professional and organized dealers benefit. For non-dealing users at the bottom of the criminal labour market, the self-financing of drug use may encourage a turn to acquisitive crime, generally of an opportunistic nature such as shoplifting, petty theft, easy burglaries. However, not all users will or can follow this path and instead may sell sexual services. At these lower levels of the criminal/drug economy we therefore see broader trends reflected – increases in property crime (and some crimes of violence) of an unsophisticated nature, committed by young people. Are we, therefore, seeing the increased participation in the drug economy of the "mass" criminal: interchangeable and unskilled, available for hire for subsistence wages, expendable to employers, immediately replaced as soon as the criminal justice system has removed one offender?

"Mass" criminals are certainly "functional" to sections of society and the legitimate economy in various ways. They create wealth which benefits ordinary customers:

> Most of these thefts materially benefit someone, either the offenders themselves, or customers who purchase stolen goods at a discounted price. . . . The aggregate benefit to low-income communities of cheaper goods is probably quite large. In the absence of such benefits, social welfare costs, which are ultimately borne by taxpayers, might rise appreciably (Greenberg 1990: 56, cf. Johnson et al. 1985).

The productivity and the wider social and economic implications of their cumulative contributions to the illicit economy are what make the "mass" criminal labour force so significant.

Our research confirms the conclusion reached by others (Mirza et al. 1991): the drug economy in London is extremely fragmented. But what has seemed to us to be worth taking further than previous accounts has been an attempt to describe the social and ethnic division of labour that can be discerned within it. This division of labour roughly reflects broader socioeconomic divisions: those employed in the drug economy who fit the category of "mass" criminals, were predominantly found in notoriously disadvantaged areas. Our findings concerning the borough of Lambeth may illustrate this point.

More than 80 per cent of the arrests for drug offences in Lambeth involve cannabis. Recidivism among cannabis offenders is very high, although the quantities of the substance seized in the area remains almost constant (Ruggiero 1993b). Many small dealers are repeat offenders, plying their trade without ever realizing any significant economic gain from it. In the words of one user, "these street dealers are there to be arrested". This is their main rôle. They are well known in the community even by those who hardly ever buy drugs. In a vicious circle and confirming a criminological truism, those who are the most penalized are also the least professional. In these cases arrest and imprisonment are not followed by criminal professionalization (but see our Turin case study below).

On the contrary, being caught and "known" decreases usefulness to employers. Limited to very low-level tasks, they are unlikely to develop any professional skills or competence. This they may often attempt to offset with simple dishonest cheating. In the words of a cannabis user in Brixton: "Here, the chances of getting oregano instead of 'grass' are very high. For this reason it's always best to have personal contacts, or to cultivate particular dealers. The most serious dealers do not live in this area".

Another user who had been in this local drug scene for the last ten years confirmed:

> Many cocaine users would come to this area to score. They think they can find anything they want here. They are usually whites who believe both the hype and the rumour that prices are lower here. They do not know, and probably they are not in a position to check, what they are getting. This also applies to cannabis. Those who come from other areas to buy cannabis make us laugh. We call the stuff they get "Brixton bush". Young people know that customers come from all over London, and of course they don't always have the good-quality stuff to sell, so they just offer what comes handy.

Our informants argued that drugs may create vast profits for someone but dealing had not stimulated their local economy, rather it was impoverished as money was taken out of the area. Given the large number of drug users in the local community, the poverty of the drug economy was interpreted as a sign that profits go to other city areas where police action is not as concentrated. Investors and large distributors were said to reside outside of central Lambeth, recruiting a number of small dealers to work for them. The implied argument is that if large distributors operated in the area, this would result in more money circulation being visible and more legitimate businesses being created with the proceeds of drug dealing. At these higher levels of drug distribution the promise of entrepreneurialism pays off but for the small dealers on the street rewards are meagre. As one drug-agency worker assessed the "professional" calibre of his clients:

132

Among my clients I don't see any Dillinger or Al Capone, but they all think they are gangsters. Somebody made them think they are – perhaps the media or the police. In fact they delude themselves: they think they are making a career, but they are just setting up the scene for themselves. They are vulnerable and obvious, they'll never make it to the top. They get nothing out of the drug economy. All they get is prison.

In the next section we shall, therefore, discuss the sociological question of why involvement in the drug economy can still be attractive.

From counterculture to enterprise-culture: drug use and dealing in London from the 1960s to the 1990s

Our description of "disadvantaged drug users" as "exploited workers" is not intended to convey the image of drug-related crime as something potentially subversive or oppositional to the social system nor to argue for special status or sympathy. On the contrary, much social harm, distress and criminal victimization can result from the illicit activities fostered by the drug economy, but it is also the case that some of these activities are remarkably similar to those pursued within the legal and productive community. Far from being "escapist" or "retreatist", these activities may reflect convention and conformity in quite striking ways. We will take this point further shortly. However, let us first see if the entrepreneurial spirit of the 1980s and 1990s is as new to drug cultures as so often assumed.

The youth cultures of the 1960s embraced behaviours, tastes, lifestyles and values which enunciated "difference" and, sometimes, declared conscious revolt. "Swinging London" was characterized by musical innovations, new tastes in fashion and style, hedonistic sociability, collective nomadism and experimentation with relationships. Of course, in reality, only a relatively small percentage of youth were aligned with political groups or fully fledged countercultures. Similarly, the extent of drug use was quite modest when compared to the 1980s and 1990s. Furthermore, although frequently associated with oppositional groups and protest, drug use also had expressive and functional value for groups that in other respects were seriously conformist – for example, the Mods who worked by day and raved at weekends, and who later metamorphosed into the suedeheads, skinheads and others whose politics were of a right-wing variety and far from sympathetic to countercultures (Redhead 1993: 2–3).

The tolerance with which the deviant young were received in the economic boom of the 1960s was partly related to their power as consumers in a rapidly changing, youth oriented market (Hall & Jefferson 1976). The symbols of "difference" and other paraphernalia (music, posters, clothes etc.) would soon become packaged commodities, as they were appropriated by industry and thrown back to their creators. While being identified as important consumers, youth also raised concern over their potential for the disruption of order. On the walls of Notting Hill slogans appeared such as: "Police Free Zone"; "I am an angry tormented soul screaming out in this torturous mediocrity"; "If voting changed anything, they'd make it illegal" (Leigh 1985). Less clearly politicized than in other European countries, rebellious youth in London distinguished themselves by the adoption of provocative lifestyles and a search for alternative artistic expressions (Frith & Horne 1987). As elsewhere in Europe, use of cannabis and LSD was common in such circles. Using these substances, or selling them, was regarded as neither immoral nor illegal. Dealers of the 1960s travelled to Lebanon and Pakistan to buy hashish: "It's the great liberating drug. Selling it isn't a business. It's more like a crusade!" (Leigh 1985: 29). Selling drugs was justifiable as part of a "freewheeling" culture which was supposed to represent an alternative to the humdrum of "straight society" and its dull rhythm, although the possibility that such an alternative might prove to bring with it its own dull routine was evident to some (Trocchi 1992). For some users, heroin was assimilated into a culture of polydrug use. Cocktails were frequent (cannabis and speed, mescaline and LSD) and some cult-novels of the early 1970s celebrated an anarchic hedonism that combined use of various drugs with a constant, unsettled search for experience and excitement (Thompson 1972).

Stewart (1987), herself an ex-heroin addict, describes these years as follows:

I acquired a tin of Golden Virginia and learnt to roll cigarettes. The lads grew their hair. Those who could grew
beards. We were into music and we followed our heroes
closely. We favoured the irreverent and anarchic: the
Stones, Dylan, Janis Joplin, the Grateful Dead, Jimi
Hendrix and the tortured Leonard Cohen. . . . They took
risks and they took drugs. The glamour and power of the
erupting volcano of rock and pop spewed out a deluge of
fine narcotic dust that threatened to cover us all (Stewart
1987: 10).

What elements of rebellion, alternative culture, solidarity and sociability are left in the behaviour of today's drug users and the drug
cultures of 1990s London? Our respondents were largely negative.
A typical statement was:

You cannot really speak of solidarity. We try to help one another all right. I try to share with my friends what I have
got. But this only happens among close friends. If you
haven't got close friends, which in London is the norm, you
are done for. Drugs, heroin in particular, make you give up
friends; everything else takes second place. After a while
you just have a relationship with the stuff and that's all.
And again, you feel bad, you are terrified that you may run
out of it. You don't care who is around you, you just care
about your stuff.

A social worker, previously employed at a central London agency
for the homeless and drug users, drew attention to what he saw as
significant changes in the social origin of his clients over the years.
In a group discussion with other social workers, he explained:

The young people we deal with now come from shattered
families. They have been given a court order, and that's
why they are in care. Some have been abused by their parents or have been abandoned. When they come here they
know they are victims, and they are convinced that society
owes them something. Some of them feel that they are entitled to a sort of revenge. They have a great need to show

their fitness for life, and in a sense they are looking for the evidence that they exist, that they have a personality. This continuing self-challenge leads them to experiment with everything, including drugs. In fact, drugs constitute a crucial passage in their search for an identity. This is nothing to do with the search for new worlds of perception, nor with a choice to be different, alternative. No rebellion is involved here. Perhaps some are lured by drugs because it is a prohibited substance. You see, they are convinced that they are not like the other ordinary people, because they are regarded as different by others. So they get used to the idea that prohibited things are the only ones suitable to them and to their condition.

Among users we interviewed many felt that the first stages of drug use encourage feelings of "being in it together", sharing and "a bit of give and take" but noted that this phase could give way to mutual suspicion, competitiveness and even aggression when drugs or money were scarce. Many complained of the stress of always having to be "on the look out" for police, other users "wanting to share your stuff", or dealers who were owed something. "Back-stabbers" were feared by both users and dealers, a situation not as common in other European cities where hierarchies seem to be more fixed and respected. One long-term user described this war of all against all very clearly:

It is so easy to get out of control. You could steal from friends or even dealers. For example, if a dealer refuses to sell on credit, he may be physically attacked. It's like an internal war, and you have to be prepared to fight it. Sometimes the attack on the dealer is planned in detail. His address is known. A couple of people who are not directly known by the dealer are picked up. In this way you grab both his stuff and his money. In cases like this the use of violence may be inevitable.

A relative scarcity of heroin on the market may ignite an all-against-all conflict, where information about dealers and their addresses are preserved with great secrecy. The terror of running out of drugs can promote a ruthless individualism. Many users contravene a code of conduct that they argue exists and routinely refuse to share drugs with others "in need". In this way they reject the basis of the "mutual society" and friendship networks that held together the social framework of user cultures in the 1960s and early 1970s. The most disheartened of our respondents claimed that the public has far less to fear from users than other users have. Most dealers take more precautions against their own underworld than against the police. They can be victimized both by users and by competing dealers. When violent episodes within the drug scene occur these may often more accurately be interpreted as simple robbery aimed at getting hold of more drugs than as territorial "turf" battles. Unsurprisingly, users suggest that it is these experiences of ceaseless hassle, competition and the absence of solidarity or honesty between users that is the main reason why they give up drugs. Many of the users we interviewed claimed that they did not like the drug scene, they just liked drugs. As Stewart (1987: 76–7) describes her ten-year experience with heroin:

> Lies are an essential part of junkiedom, at first, to protect yourself from the obvious consequences of heroin, later, to avoid having to share your drugs with someone else. Junkies become suspicious of one another and they are sharp-eyed. . . . A junkie who has been turned away by someone he knows will wait until that person is sick and go round just to chase gear in front of him.

Among our London informants the cocaine market was generally seen as even more conducive to commercialization and thus to heavy competition. In the view of one drug worker: "Cocaine may constitute a realistic career choice – more so than other drugs. It is true that there are probably still some old-style bohemian-type cocaine dealers, who use the substance and share it with their peers. But in general, commercial relationships prevail in the cocaine market and very ambitious individuals force their way into it. For these reasons, perhaps the cocaine underworld is more problematic".

Gender relations in the drug economy

Traditional values and practices can also be seen in the drug economy when we consider the treatment of women. Opinions and research findings on this subject differ, the available literature being mainly polarized by two perspectives. In the first perspective the rôle of women in the drug underworld is assumed to be a passive one, a rôle also involving victimization. The second perspective ascribes an active rôle to female drug users, whose subjectivity and free choice is emphasized. To illustrate the first perspective, McRobbie (1980) has noted how the rituals and mythologies attached to heroin and other drug use are so narrowly male that few women feel any interest in them. One reason for this is said to reside in "the commonsense wisdom deeply inscribed in most women's consciousnesses – that boys don't like girls who drink, take speed and so on; that losing control spells sexual danger; and that drinking and taking drugs harm physical appearance" (ibid.: 46).

Similarly, Rosenbaum (1982) observes that "women on heroin" have been termed "damaged commodities", stigmatized both by law abiding people and by their male user counterparts (cf. Taylor 1993). Women are judged on their appearance more than men, and once the routine of keeping up a supply of heroin is underway, little time and money are left for keeping up one's appearance (Stewart 1987). Most of our male respondents said they did not like to see "girls on heroin", "there's no glamour or mystery in it". The majority of the female users they knew had come into contact with heroin because their partners were users before them. Some women get involved in the heroin scene in order to protect their men who have already acquired a criminal record. They then resolve to "hustle" rather than put their partners at risk of re-offending and therefore re-conviction (cf. Taylor 1993, Chs. 2 and 3, on women heroin users in Glasgow).

Tradition and conformity are also detectable in relationships where the male heroin user, wittingly or otherwise, expects his partner to perform a rôle of nurse or social worker. This is particularly the case when attempts, or gestures, at "coming off" are made by men, a circumstance that "gives males an emotional lever of use to them in their dealing with women" (Auld et al. 1986: 177, McRobbie 1980). The inexhaustible female is then supposed to provide her male partner with emotional and material services, while thinking that she has both beaten her "chemical rival" and shattered the barrier of toughness previously built by her man.

> It is not difficult to see what a young man may get out of this: refreshed, fed, and wearing clean clothes, he rises and goes back on the street, having had the type of "holiday" that sexual divisions provide a young man "working" in the irregular economy. A whole series of episodic cycles of consumption of heroin and of girlfriend-assisted "coming-off" may follow. All aspects of the cycle – work, consumption, and the temporary retirement from and rejuvenation of masculinity – may be enjoyable in their ways (Auld et al. 1986: 179).

From a different perspective, substance abuse for women has been regarded as a challenge to traditional female stereotypes and rôles related to the identity of a "real" woman (Perry 1979, Ettorre 1989, 1992). Specifically, it is argued that female drug users and dealers are the epitome of women who fail to conform to the official values commonly attributed to femininity. "In reality, she is a non-woman in the public sphere and her visibility is a direct challenge to the established patriarchal order" (Ettorre 1989: 106). Subjectivity and choice are also invoked by authors who claim that among the reasons why women enter the drug scene is the perception that it provides an expansion of life options (Rosenbaum & Murphy 1990). Women are attracted to drugs, it is argued, because they want to be part of a social scene that offers "the appearance (and sometimes the reality) of money, excitement, and the euphoric properties of drugs" (ibid.: 121–2).

The common assumption that women are introduced to heroin through male acquaintances or friends has often proved wrong according to studies in the USA (Gerkin et al. 1977, Rosenbaum 1981, Waldorf 1973) and with some anecdotal support for Britain. Many women frequently start their using career through legal prescriptions of pharmaceuticals as they attempt to alleviate physical pain and psychological distress. They eventually turn to the illicit market when prescriptions run out or are withdrawn by doctors (Prather & Fidell 1978). The notion that women who take drugs are passive victims of circumstances has also been challenged. A study conducted in Merseyside concluded that taking drugs may provide women with an alternative to a life of apathy and powerlessness, in that it initially promises excitement, purpose, and a structure for daily action (Buchanan et al. 1991). Contrary to images of women as irrational, pathological and passive, most female users claimed that they were not dependent on men for their supply, and they "were quite explicit that their offending was not due to irrational behaviour or emotional problems" (ibid.: 61).

Whether passive victims or enterprising actors, women who enter the drug scene often find a reflection, if not an exacerbation, of the rôle divisions operating in society as a whole. Vulnerable to threats and violence they may themselves become victims of acquisitive crime committed by male users (Ruggiero 1993b). A woman manager of a drug project in South London suggested that many of the women users she deals with are forced into prostitution by the "conservatism" of the drug scene:

> Prostitution re-establishes sex roles within a setting that one would think less conservative than the official society. The sex industry in this country is now bigger than it's ever been. Some female drug users continue their career as prostitutes even after coming off drugs. This is degrading and dangerous, and explains how people who most suffer the consequences of drug-related crime are users themselves, especially those most vulnerable.

Women drug users are stigmatized both by the general public and by their own male peers. In many cases they are also exploited by their male counterparts. We met a number of "bag-followers", who were looked down upon for their dependence on drugs and on someone else to provide them. We also met individual women who felt they had certainly fulfilled the rôle of exploited "nurse" and provided emotional and material services for their partners for little reward. Several "independent" female heroin users with whom we made contact were strongly disapproved of because they were seen as neglecting their children. Others were alternatively valued or shunned because of their prostitution.

Internationally, the exploitation of women in the drug economy is manifest in their employment as cross-border couriers (Green 1991). Exploitation and stereotyping are also apparent in the crimes that women may be expected to undertake; for example, women are often given the task of shop-lifting because it is assumed they will be less noticeable and less suspicious as shoppers than men. They pay a higher toll for their addiction socially and often in terms of penal response (Worral 1990, Bild & Hayes 1992). The drug user life can also be heavier for women than for men in other ways: "Women may suffer physically more than men, which can present problems concerning presentation of self. Daily drug use often causes premature ageing. Women appear older and worn out, while their male counterparts seem to recuperate easily" (Rosenbaum & Murphy 1990: 122).

Overall, the position of women in the drug underworld does not differ from the position of women in general: blocked in criminal careers as they are in legal ones.

Conclusion: recent and future trends in the London drug market

Current drug use trends suggest that polydrug use is the predominant pattern in the early 1990s (ISDD/Ashton 1993: 7). Within this pattern there may be various developments of interest. One would seem to be the extent to which the police are effectively decriminalizing possession of cannabis in small amounts, at least for a first offence and in some circumstances. A second is that cocaine and crack seem to be at the dynamic edge of the ever-changing drugs market. This is not to say that the dark and pessimistic prophesies of the 1980s, which suggested that Britain would soon be awash with crack and coke, are about to be fulfilled. It is to suggest that in parts of London, as in other cities in the UK, availability of cocaine and crack is rising, and profits, criminal organization and violence are not unexpected accompaniments. Further research on just who the "new cocaine and crack users" are, and what services are available or needed, might be useful. Certainly the picture so far is quite mixed (Mott 1992, Dean et al. 1992, Ditton et al. 1991, Bean 1993).

How far the incidence of violence in drug related crime is actually increasing and how far media fed concerns have magnified the problem is unclear. Nonetheless, the issue of firearms use is an important one to monitor in Britain and it may be possible to argue that some of the currently unproductive police time expended on small-scale drugs offences could be better directed towards preventing the further development of a different illegal market – that for guns. Gun control could become a significant item on the law enforcement agenda in the 1990s with benefits in terms of slowing the process of arming the police and reducing certain attractions and dangers in the drug trade (Kaletsky 1993).

However, cocaine and crack, and related anxieties about violence etc., must not capture all the attention of policy and practice. The reality of cannabis as the most popular illegal drug in the capital and the rest of the UK and Europe, makes its continued criminal status increasingly anomalous. Does Amsterdam's tolerance policy of decriminalization, not legalization, offer some kind of blueprint for London and other European cities? (See Chapter 3). Legalization or decriminalization of heroin in a regulated commercial market is a far less likely prospect and here harm-minimization principles should continue to underpin social work and health practice (South 1993), (although some government ministers have recently questioned this approach in an ominous way; Druglink 1993: 5). Certainly intravenous use of opiates has not gone away (Mirza et al. 1991: 6.1), despite high profile educational campaigns about AIDS/HIV (Dorn & South 1991b, Power 1989). ISDD's 1992 Drug Misuse Audit observed that at the end of 1991 the purity of heroin had increased to 47 per cent, a rise from 35–40 per cent the year before and 30 per cent in 1987, while seizures were also rising – developments interpreted "by enforcement authorities" as "evidence of heroin's increased availability and popularity" (ISDD/ Ashton 1993: 9, 15).

Overall, data from the Thames Region Drug Misuse Databases (Daniel 1993: 71) offer a snapshot of problem drug use known to agencies in Greater London at the beginning of the 1990s, as follows:

> In Greater London as a whole, nearly eight thousand (7978) individuals were reported as presenting to services between 1st April 1991 and 31st March 1992. . . . The inci-

dence of presenting drug users was notably higher in some inner London areas, where rates of over 7 per 1000 were found, while in Bloomsbury and Islington the rate was over 1 per hundred . . .

A high incidence of heroin use was noted across the London region. Over half of episodes (5299) reported to the databases involved heroin as the primary drug. Methadone was the second most commonly reported main drug, although reports were lower at 16% (1389) of the total.

Use of cocaine, benzodiazepines, cannabis and amphetamines as main drugs was less widespread, accounting respectively for 4.2%, 5.5% and 2.8% of reports. Use of these substances as secondary drugs was much higher, suggesting their importance in polydrug use, and in particular, the trend for primary opiate users to supplement or combine other drugs.

Health and HIV

The situation may change, but some note must be made of the high concentration of drug-related HIV and AIDS cases in the London area. This bears upon the issue of harm minimization and the shaping of future behaviours among drug users, approaches and co-ordination of helping services, and the issue of balancing enforcement targeting of the drug market with health oriented, anti-HIV initiatives. The necessity of taking these matters seriously in the 1990s is underlined by the experiences of the 1980s and the correlation of high HIV rates with punitive policies, as in Edinburgh, and low rates and liberal policies, as in Merseyside. As Pearson & Gilman (1994: 111) summarize:

Levels of known HIV infection among injecting drug users in the British Isles show marked regional variations. In England, almost two-thirds of known cases are to be found in the greater London area. Moreover, as many as 30% of all English reports come from the single regional health authority of North West Thames. The most marked regional variation, however, is that between Scotland and the rest of the United Kingdom. Of all HIV antibody positive reports in the United Kingdom among drug injectors to the end of 1990, 44% were to be found in Scotland. On this basis, greater London accounts for approximately one-third of reports of HIV infection in the entire UK. By contrast, less than 1% of such reports came from the Merseyside region.

Developments in the Greater London area often (though not always) presage developments elsewhere. In this respect, while we would not support the London-centrism that has often dominated British drug-related social policy in the past, the case can be made that continued attention to trend data and ethnographic studies relating to epidemiology, HIV and other drug issues in London, may pay dividends in illuminating trends nationally.

5

Heroin use and distribution in Turin: politics and rebels, commodities and entrepreneurs

Turin: the origin of heroin use

Throughout the 1960s, visible and lively countercultures flourished in Turin but a specific drug culture was largely – and surprisingly – absent. In the account of one veteran user:

> I recall that in 1966 a French guy arrived from Marseille with some heroin of excellent quality: well, he didn't manage to sell any. Thinking about it, a real and distinctive cannabis culture did not exist either. Around the same time, a friend brought a kilo of kif (hashish oil) from Morocco, and he couldn't sell it either.

Without an established market to ensure supply, regular cannabis users were obliged to provide for themselves by undertaking repeated trips to Morocco. The quantity of cannabis purchased and the amount of money spent, were shared among friends and acquaintances, who constituted a consortium of equal members. The distribution system extended throughout this friendship and peer network. In time, more expensive and adventurous trips were undertaken by "sponsored" groups or simply by those who had more time and travelling experience. Good quality kif could be bought in India and Afghanistan – all that was required was the expenditure of a little more money and willingness to take a slightly bigger risk.

The first serious users of opiate type drugs also found they could not rely on supply via an established illicit market and instead resorted to pharmaceutical sources:

> We would forge prescriptions and buy morphine. Another very common drug for some time, was cardiostenolo, which could be injected. As a substitute to morphine, a tablet called talwin would frequently be bought. This, in fact, does not produce a great deal of a high, unless it is taken in huge quantities. However it was easily available in any pharmacy.

Talwin rapidly became a favourite drug in the early 1970s, despite its modest performance as a euphoric agent or pain killer. This has been explained in terms of other properties of the drug:

> Talwin pills would simulate the "transgressive'"game of fixing, they were fit for social gatherings, they were convivial. Very cheap and available without any risk, everybody would offer it to everybody. It did not stone completely, but it gave a temporary feeling of well being. Talwin would also be used in large quantities, and eventually abused, in order to avoid the use of other hard drugs (D'Este 1990: 92).

Travel to India also provided access to an unanticipated source of opiate supply – over-spill from the legitimate international pharmaceutical trade in such drugs. Users reported being able to purchase large quantities of very cheap morphine tablets, which were provided by the German firm Bayer as part of medical aid for India and other Third World countries. Those who specifically wanted heroin would travel to Amsterdam, both on their own account and as representatives of groups of users. In the early 1970s:

> The variety *brown sugar* was available in Amsterdam, and its success was perhaps due to the cult-song of The Rolling Stones which had the same title. Using hard drugs was part of this counter-culture, it entailed an alternative life-style to the official society. Nothing like the heroin users of today. Nothing to do with profits. (user-dealer).

Rather more than in the UK and some other European countries, the Italian countercultures of the 1960s and the 1970s were distinguished by a high degree of politicization. This explains why so many early heroin users in Italy were members of grass-roots political organizations.

> In Turin in particular, the first users were political militants of the left. They were not addicted to heroin, but occasional consumers who saw in heroin a symbol and a practice of rebellion. Therefore it is not surprising that even today, among users and dealers, people who were previously very committed politically can be found in large numbers. And this is also why, if you come from a similar political background it is easy to contact them, discuss with them and often achieve a common understanding. (ex-user)

This picture was confirmed by a middle-range distributor in Turin who is still operating in the market and who boasted of his long and complex career. Although outside the political culture of the time and distanced from its strong ideological principles, this dealer nonetheless shared the attitudes and lifestyle of the early users. This does not have to sound paradoxical. In some sections of the extreme left, rejection of official society and of conformist behaviour was so firm that the search for "different" behaviour would also be pursued within the illegal sphere. In this context, natural allies would also be sought among those who, whether bereft of ideology or because of it, practised illegality as a daily economic activity. The encounter between these two illegalities, one of an *occupational* character, the other, of a *political* nature, occurred in Turin at the end of the 1960s. This encounter gave birth to groups which eventually became known in town under the name of *comontisti* (a local variant of highly politicized Situationists). One point needs stressing about such groups: although of militant character they are not to be confused with other political organizations (the *Red Brigades* and the *Nuclei Armati Proletari*) that, in subsequent years, targeted the "lumpen proletariat" with the aim of raising their political consciousness.

It is interesting to see how this encounter between two different arenas of illegal activity is recalled by participants from this period.

The following is a typical account of a non-politicized person:

> Yes, I have a criminal record, I have been arrested several
> times. The first time for car theft, when I was still under
> eighteen. I have also been charged with armed robbery and
> kidnapping. This latter charge involved a political abduc-
> tion carried out against the boss of a mechanic firm in Tu-
> rin. I had connections with people of the left. Years ago this
> mixture of different people was frequent, especially in
> groups like the *comontisti*. I was not a political person, but I
> did things with them from time to time. *We would share
> smack and hang around together. They were politically very ac-
> tive, they would not only reject society as a whole but also any
> form of hierarchical organization and all forms of authority.
> They theorised illegality both because they were a bit romantic
> and perhaps because many comontisti had a criminal record
> anyway, and lived on petty crime.* (emphasis added)

In the same vein:

> It was fun with the *comontisti*. There was no lack of money,
> we would go out, to restaurants and clubs, we would get
> stoned, no problem. It was not like now, in that even if you
> used heroin you were not a *junkie*. We would just enjoy our-
> selves, like ordinary people. Of course we would shoplift or
> do little robberies. We felt free and were disgusted by "re-
> spectable" people and their boring life.

One of the founders of these groups, who is still politically active,
gives a more detached account:

> The *comontisti* occupied the most extreme sector of the po-
> litical spectrum. We were profoundly libertarian and we
> adopted non-Leninist revolutionary groups such as the
> Makhnovists among our ideological models (anarchist
> Machno and his followers were very active during the So-
> viet revolution). A slogan coined in those years went:
> Against Capital the Fight Must Be Criminal (Lotta
> criminale contro il capitale). Very radical, unsettled, indi-

vidualistic, we criticized official politics as a whole and were scathing against those who saw politics as a profession, both on the right and on the left. Highly ideologised and culturally very lively (we would devour books and ideas coming from all over the world), we were the first heroin users in Turin.

The coexistence of highly politicized users alongside individuals involved in conventional illegality lasted until the first organized groups moved into the heroin market of Turin. This event, in turn, was perceived by the two groups in a different manner. The "politicized", who were by now accustomed to alternating use of cannabis, pharmaceuticals and heroin, suddenly found it very difficult to get hold of anything but heroin. Now it was this drug that dominated the market and prices rose abruptly: "Some groups of distributors started to impose market prices. A dose, which was bought in Amsterdam for 20.000 lire (£10), would be sold in Turin for 70–80.000. Distribution was carried out by small groups of criminals previously only involved in robberies". (cf. our account of the emergence of criminal distributors in London).

The criminal, "non-politicized" groups simply saw heroin distribution as an "innovation" in their career. Those routinely involved in theft and robbery who had mixed with the comontisti (without sharing their ideology), interpreted the changing market as a logical evolution: the orientation of illegal activities towards a more profitable and less risky business was simply a natural development. Among these small-scale criminals, those who had used and were familiar with heroin, also aimed to capitalize on its increasing commercial value. At this time – the early to mid 1970s – the market did not yet resemble the conventional picture of mafia-style organized crime, but instead involved relatively small groups who were still independent in their operations and who were moving away from their previous activities and shifting into a new one. A dealer recalls:

> I would go to Amsterdam myself. I already knew the scene up there because I had done business with the comontisti. I would be given some money by five or six people who wanted to invest it. Those who had more money were the small groups of armed robbers who clearly sensed the ad-

vantages of the new business. Everything suddenly seemed very easy. There was no need to risk one's life any more, it finally seemed the end of guns. That was an amazing and unique period. New businesses were created, some of these ex-robbers would buy a restaurant or a club, or even a luxury shop in the centre of town. Some of them, after a couple of operations, would finally retire and set up a "clean" business. Some would do both, invest in heroin from time to time, and still keep their clean business going. (cf. the categories of "diversifying criminals" and "sideliners" discussed earlier.)

Some groups of users reacted to the commercial shift and creation of a tougher market, in quite the opposite way. The new "business dealers" were first threatened and eventually confronted with violence. These new distributors were disapproved of not for being drug dealers but for being entrepreneurs. In the words of an ex-user:

It is one thing to pay for one's expenses and perhaps make a living, it is another thing to set up an industry and become a capitalist. This was our reasoning, one (which was) certainly very ideological and candid and which would currently sound laughable. Nevertheless one could look nostalgically to that period and that "naive" attitude. The comontisti acted as a sort of "social service", as they tried to prevent the first heroin traders from creating a new generation of customers. Against the new distributors a number of punitive actions were carried out.

The local newspapers erroneously recorded these "punitive actions" as episodes of internal struggle between dealers' gangs fighting for dominance in the market. Instead, they were part of a naïve battle against changes which were already too far advanced to be turned around. Nonetheless, such actions did, in time, have some effect on the way that distribution developed in Turin. In the centre of town, where "aware" users had established their social space and market, heroin was subjected to prudent price-control due to the negotiating power of the "politicized". In the peripheral areas of the town, where high levels of demand were anticipated, distribution was soon decentralized and prices almost doubled. In a short while however, both the users and the independent groups of distributors were faced with the entry of organized crime into the heroin market, coinciding with the emergence of a new key figure: the non-user distributor.

To summarize: between the 1960s and the early 1970s heroin use in Turin involved stark generational conflicts and is best understood in terms of the feelings of discontent that were expressed in the political movements born in 1968 (Merlo 1988). In Italy, it could be argued that heroin use was one of the elements, if extreme and circumscribed, of such political expression.

The phases of heroin use

Respondents found it difficult to decide whether the increase in heroin use in Turin, from the 1960s on, was simply due to an increase in availability or whether other factors were involved. It is of course, difficult to be sure of the accuracy and degree of self-justification in recollections tinged by nostalgia and stretching back around twenty years. But certainly, the development of a heroin "epidemic" in Turin was attributed to the networking of peers and friends: the first offer of heroin usually coming from a close and trustworthy person. Some recalled periods when certain drugs were being given a "promotional push", as when suddenly, and for several months, cannabis was impossible to find on the market, which was then suspiciously flooded with heroin, giving rise to "conspiracy theories" about planned market manipulation.

Among the early heroin users in Turin, only a few became addicted and none seem to have overdosed or contracted Aids. The use of heroin as simply a part of a broader set of social and political acts may have diminished the power of the drug and encouraged use on an intermittent and transitory basis. An early user, who eventually gave up heroin to devote all his energies to anti-institutional politics, remarked:

> Then [in the late 1970s] the users from the destitute suburbs came on the scene. They were the real novelty. Distri-

bution became thorough, decentralized, every area of town had its outlets. The organizations became efficient, structured as an industry. Heroin became a mass commodity like any other commodity. The users' culture obviously also changed. The new users did not have cultural defences, they could not self-manage heroin use. Completely different performances and effects were demanded from heroin by these new users as compared to the politicised ones. They were certainly more vulnerable not only in the face of heroin, but in the face of all commodities. . . . They were incapable of controlling the nature, the quality, the quantity and the use-value of the substance.

Heroin no longer provided a symbol for collective political identity. Instead recreational use became dominant, displacing other activities in which the users had been involved: "When heroin use becomes a rite, it gives the unrepeatable pleasure of a total transgression. The users feel that they are completely 'out'. No pleasure could be more intense for adolescents than the awareness of being out of everything, against everybody" (Gallo et al. 1980: 13)

A clear snapshot of some of the features of this second phase of heroin use is provided by a piece of research conducted on behalf of the Health Authority of the Piedmont Region in 1979. This study noted that although occasional users had constituted the majority in the previous phase, they now accounted for only 2 per cent of the heroin using population known to the official agencies. About 90 per cent injected heroin daily and more than once a day (Assessorato alla Sanita', 1980). The quantitative scale of drug addiction was the most striking development of the period between 1975–80. In this phase, problematic use spread significantly among 18–25 year olds, just at the time when the heroin under-world was losing its associations with a past of political and rebellious motivation.

Commentators remarked on the relative youth of heroin users, few being above 30: "This can partly be explained by the fact that heroin arrived in Turin in relatively recent years [1973–4]. However this also seems to confirm that in the course of their heroin use career the addicts achieve a relative stability and integration within society, as they either stop habitual use or learn to self-manage use of the substance" (Magistratura Democratica 1980: 52). This conclusion suggests that heroin use in Turin soon became adapted to ordinary, non-political lifestyles.

Nonetheless, throughout the 1970s, there still lingered a "cultural trace" left over from the previous phase of heroin use. At public discussions in Turin between 1977–80, groups of heroin users presented themselves as formally organized, campaigning for the legalization of drugs and emulating the practices and slogans of those more politicized groups still active. A leaflet distributed at one conference declared: "The Health authority, nurses and doctors must stand clear of us. We deny anybody the right to make judgements about our choices, and will do our best to escape from those like you who want to study and analyze us in your poisoning laboratories" (quoted in Gallo et al. 1980).

Groups of specialist social workers supported their clients in similar campaigns. They were also formally organized and deeply involved in "deconstructing" the official label of heroin addiction. For example, their refusal to regard heroin use as a pathology was presented as a formal statement:

> A total medicalization of life is underway which is transforming every citizen into a patient or a potential patient. Physiological states of being tend to be assimilated to moments of risk; in turn, all human ages become "risk ages", whereby specialised surveillance is required on everybody. Soon we will all have to delegate our autonomy to the therapists (*Il Manifesto*, 7 November 1979).

A similar view was expressed in another leaflet:

> Heroin use in the Western Countries is depicted with a demonic and deadly nature that it does not possess. But this false image acts as a device which diverts attention from the deadly reality of industrial systems: cancer, pollution, etc. On the other hand, the image of the heroin addict creates social consensus, as it persuades public opinion of the utility of repressive institutions such as the police, of professionals such as the psychiatrists, and of all the petit-bourgeois who vent their frustrations upon the deviants (Gallo et al. 1980).

In many detoxification centres, staff and clients found that they shared a common past and similar political experiences. The detoxification centres had been established in Turin in 1978 and many "militant" professionals regarded their clients as underprivileged users, in contrast to others who could afford therapy in private clinics (Bonino 1982). Rehabilitation was an idea viewed with caution because it was seen as intrinsically moralistic. The empathy of the social workers and doctors from the detoxification centres is also reflected in the reporting of heroin addiction. All cases known to the city's juvenile court were reported by the police or families and private citizens – not one case of drug addiction was notified by the detoxification centres! (Magistratura Democratica 1980).

A third phase of heroin use developed from around 1980 to 1985 (Censis 1986). In Turin, this phase saw a yearly increase of 600 known heroin addicts: between 1979 and 1982 cases rose from 1298 to 3234. The increase would later settle at an average 300 cases per year, while the number of officially known heroin addicts would reach 4160 in 1985 (Regione Piemonte 1985). By now, observers assumed that the public drugs agencies were in contact with only a limited proportion of the new heroin users. For example, only one-third of the addicts incarcerated were known to the detoxification centres before their arrest (ibid.). Those clients that the centres did see had diverse social characteristics. Research conducted by the local health authority found that 40 per cent of clients were either employed or "under-employed", many were students and very few were unemployed, save those who became so after developing a heroin habit and/or after arrest.

In this third phase, heroin users in Turin reflected diversity rather than community and cultural fragmentation rather than the solidarity of shared experience. These users were part of different groups more distant from one another than from "straight" official society. Here there were:

> old members of the "new left" who are undergoing a phase of political disorientation, new 'rebels' who have been bred on "alternative" music, the thirty-somethings who resort to heroin after years of alcoholism and tabagism (nicotine addiction), and the very young who wear designer clothes, use expensive perfumes and buy "Timberland" shoes (Rinascita, 10 February 1984).

In drug cultures reflecting isolation rather than solidarity, older users no longer transmitted information and advice to younger novices: "Information about the nature and the effects of drugs is absolutely lacking. Many young people claim that they have shifted from hashish to heroin, as they thought the new substance was only different in the administration technique rather than in the nature and effects" (Bonino 1982: 236).

It was in this same period that a national directive on treatment ruled that methadone should now be administered orally rather than allowing the previous practice of injecting it. It is hard to assess how much impact this directive had on the growth of heroin addiction but certainly the abrupt change pushed some users towards the illicit market and dissuaded neophytes from contacting the detoxification centres (cf. the British experience described earlier). Some associated the policy with the increasing stigmatization of heroin users:

> Some years ago we would get methadone from the detox centres, but we were trusted as to how and when we used it. We would be given a certain quantity to use, and dose according to personal needs. Some used to take a dose in the morning, before going to work, so that a normal active day could ensue. Then this new rule was introduced that methadone had to be administered and consumed in the centres themselves, on the premises, under the supervision of a doctor or a social worker. Moreover, the centres are now only open at certain hours of the day, and we have to be there at precise times. Hence, we can't have an ordinary life, but we are expected to act like heroin addicts, like patients who see their doctor every day. In this way we are very visible and immediately identifiable. If I wanted, as you say, to "cohabit" with heroin, and lead an ordinary life with it, I could no longer do it.

Research surveying Turin pharmacists at this time indicated that 3000 syringes were sold daily to heroin users and simultaneously that there was a notable increase in the quantity of psychotropes purchased (Merlo 1988: 50).

In the most recent phase of heroin use 1985-93, a pattern of polydrug use has developed. Now consumption of licit pharmaceutical drugs may be mixed with, substituted for, or alternated with heroin use. In this period it became evident that some users were attempting to reconcile their drug use with an ordinary daily life. So-called "transition youths" tried to ensure that their drug using career was compatible with the adult world of work and responsibility (Radio Flash and Radio Torino Popolare 1989). It is mostly with this phase that the following section is concerned.

The consumers

The new drug users are aware that they represent wide-spread socioeconomic differences and cultural diversity. Only for the most disadvantaged is heroin use associated with and disapproved of as "drug addiction". Here we provide examples of the whole range of users.

Users belonging to upper and middle-class social groups are usually resented by others because of the way they use heroin as a luxury item:

> In Turin there are very respectable places to score where only selected customers are admitted. This is the case with chic bars and clubs, where people like me would not be allowed. These places are frequented by wealthy people who can buy all sorts of drugs in a very discreet environment. There you find good quality cocaine, but heroin is also bought. Moreover, the wealthy users can afford to smoke or sniff heroin because the quality they get is pure.

Such resentment is compounded by the unequal distribution of stigma and shame – people may use the same drug but be treated in very different ways by society. As in London, there is a growing overlap between markets for cocaine and heroin, where familiarity with the former may entice someone into experimentation with the latter, although it is significant that in these circles both substances are either smoked or inhaled thus distancing their use from associations with injecting and marginalization. At the same time, heroin is used by some wealthy cocaine users to temper the cocaine "buzz".

In recent years the use of drug cocktails has been expanding and today the market offers a variety of drugs for a variety of lifestyles. These cocktails are compatible with both productive behaviour and recreational activities. Moreover, they do not carry the stigma of association with the junkie lifestyle. Some respondents suggested that drugs of the future will adapt to mass tastes and consumption and will replicate, as it were, the history of other consumer-products such as cars. At first, luxury items are scarce and reserved for the elite, after a while they are available in compact economy versions for everybody. According to other opinions, the idea that there will be a convergence of drug use between upper and middle-classes and the lower classes is inconceivable. A very clear view of the strength of social class divisions and the differentiation of drugs and their users was held by most social workers interviewed. As one of them astutely noted:

It is true that the socially privileged users can afford high quality drugs. But we cannot predict whether a massification and uniformity of available drugs is in progress. A market for wealthy drug users makes sense only if a parallel market exists where the quality is awful and where the stereotypes hold sway. It will always be useful to identify an "evil" drug which confirms the identity of those who reject it.

Further down the class structure, users from diverse occupational sectors are found. Heroin use in Turin involves (in varying measure) workers employed in the tertiary sector, factories, part-time and occasional workers, the unemployed, petty criminals, and current and ex-prisoners. Here are some examples of the different categories.

I have worked in publicity as a designer. I am now self-employed and work at home, I draw cartoons. I have been using heroin for 7–8 years and I have stopped from time to time for short periods. Nobody ever forced me to stop, I just wanted to do something else, like enjoying other things that I usually have no time to appreciate. I am talking about simple things: going to the seaside, but also meeting different people than the ones I hang around with, concentrating on my work a bit more, basically get some satisfaction out of life. These are the motivations which now and again make me stop.

This informant and others suggested that intermittent heroin use is only possible if users have access to other social groups. Many claimed to "control" the substance although using it daily, because they were still attracted or stimulated by other tasks (e.g. their employment) and by human relationships (colleagues, friends) (cf. Zinberg 1984, Blackwell 1983). Of course, some users may shift from habitual to occasional use and back again, during careers which can span a decade or more, and combine a heroin using "career" with a normal occupational career.

Heroin use in Turin also spread in traditional occupational sectors generally characterized by strong co-worker solidarity and socialization. In many cases, respondents suggested that the heroin lifestyle could become a substitute for the work milieu, the latter no longer providing an environment that stimulated common interests or collective politics. In fact, dissatisfaction with work, not the lack of it, was one reason given for heroin experimentation. Even in the factories of Turin, where traditionally the working class has found a source of political identity and strength, individualism and competing aspirations may overshadow common material and political interests.

> Even at work, they all keep to themselves. One has to find pretexts to do something together or even to talk. I don't ask anybody to discuss matters with me because I feel embarrassed, let alone asking someone to meet after work. So, an appointment with somebody to score heroin and fix it together provides an artificial excuse to have company and it makes you feel that you have got a common task with someone. Of course, after a while you only know people who fix and start missing people who don't. You get bored talking all the time with people like you who score and fix, you would like to be stimulated by other sorts of people . . . but how?

That heroin use involves individuals from diverse social backgrounds was illustrated over a matter of 30 hours between the 27 and the 28 October 1988. During this period, 6 young people died in Turin of a heroin overdose: one of them was the son of a small entrepreneur, one was a civil servant, another a lorry driver, two were industrial workers, and one unemployed. The whole occupational spectrum of the town was represented. It might be that the inexperience of several of these overdose victims made them particularly vulnerable, insofar as they might have little idea what they were buying and their tolerance for additives or higher than usual purity levels would be limited. This is partly true but, more fundamentally, the deaths can be attributed to the way the market was operating (a subject we shall deal with in more depth later). The key point is that the market at this time was also attracting inexperienced dealers, whose skills in testing the strength of heroin and cutting it appropriately were quite limited. In this respect, respondents observed that occasional users are very vulnerable in that they have difficulties managing the effects of heroin.

Some overdose deaths that have been officially categorised as "suicides" have also been interpreted as representing an extreme manifestation of impotence and despair. Such suicides are also held to indicate that some users, while wanting to give up heroin use, do not see any viable alternative. In the area of Turin called Mirafiori, roughly half of the heroin deaths over the last few years are attributed to the deliberate intent of the user to "put an end to it" through a premeditated dosage error.

Further down the local social hierarchy, heroin users are found who become familiar with the drug while involved in routine illegal activities and those who experiment with it in prison. A dealer with several experiences of prison life, observed:

> the moral taboo connected to heroin use is easily broken in prison. There, many try heroin for the first time, perhaps due to their desperate condition in the cell. Once they learn how to use it, and once they get to know it properly, they also become accustomed to the idea of selling it. Some are a bit scared at the beginning, but then they start appreciating it. I took some heroin into prison that was not detected in my body when I was arrested. Well, I had to face a queue: "give me some of that tisane", they would say. Before being imprisoned these people had no idea what heroin was.

For this type of new user, the encounter with heroin very often entails moving away from the illegal activities in which they were previously involved. It also means their subjection both to heroin and to a criminal group which guarantees its provision:

> The conditions of heroin users who work for a criminal organization are very heavy. Those who accept the role are forced to act as toughly and to be as ruthless as their bosses act with them. If they deal with me, for example, they realize that I don't have a criminal record like theirs, that I am not part of their world. So they regard me as a petit bourgeois who takes heroin for kicks and whose life is easy.

An assessment of heroin use in Italy would not be complete without considering users in institutional settings. This does not necessarily just mean those who are "on the wrong side of the law" and imprisoned. Recent reports have suggested that heroin use is also spreading in the police service and that some officers, after experimenting with the substance, quickly "leap" into selling it (*La Repubblica*, 22 March 1990). Such episodes were reported in Bologna and Milan, and more recently also in Turin. (New York also has a long tradition of such re-cycling of drugs back onto the street with a Mayoral Commission hearing evidence of another such scandal in 1993). Our respondents provided similar examples from their own experience. It was also suggested that in some anti-drugs police operations, an overlap of rôles and the unclear distribution of functions within the force make it very difficult to keep track of all the drugs seized and some may be diverted for personal use and/or resale. Moreover, it was suggested that because undercover officers often tolerate small-scale dealing in order to trace connections between street and middle-range distribution, they become vulnerable to corruption and the temptation to engage in some buying and selling on their own account. After recent judicial investigations, a group of prison officers were sentenced for providing heroin to the inmates of "Le Nuove" prison in Turin. One of them claimed to have been coerced into the distribution business by threats made by "powerful" prisoners. Another asserted that he had experimented with heroin use at work because it simply "was around" and because it provided relief from stress. Having become a user, he saw nothing wrong in distributing the substance to prisoners who were also users (*La Stampa*, 16 June 1989, *La Repubblica*, 8 May 1990). But what happened to the old users? To those hyper-politicized initiators of heroin use who saw conformists, not heroin addicts, as "the living dead" and who coined the slogan: "let death find us alive"? The answer is that most of them simply gave up: they retain a spirit of defiance but can now only manage pessimistic denunciations of the system.

> I think that all the attempts, more or less genuinely motivated, to fight against drugs are very naïve. It is like fighting against cars, whose production is inexorable in spite of the enormous social costs involved in car production. Both in the case of cars and hard drugs the industry is so strong that the product becomes necessary. Nobody wonders, when buying a car, whether that car is going to kill them. The same happens with hard drugs: everybody knows that their quality is appalling, that it can be lethal, but this does not prevent them from buying it. Experimental use and self-management of heroin are no longer possible. We are just faced with a situation where a customer purchases a commodity in a supermarket and where in spite of the apparent freedom of choice there exists a condition of slavery and monopoly.

Residual rebellion or perpetuating conformity?

In Italy today, heroin use and the "heroin culture" are frequently associated with marginalization and social inequality and, in these circumstances, heroin use may still signify an act representing some form of rebellion, triggered by the experience of social conditions that leave many unfulfilled: "To be young in Turin means to be on average less satisfied with oneself, with the town, with one's leisure time. It also means being more lonely than the other young people living in other cities of North Italy" (Ricolfi et al. 1988: 152).

It could be argued that a residual form of rebellion is alive among the disadvantaged youth who use heroin, in that they seek to distance themselves from a society that glamorizes wealth but excludes them from access to legitimate luxuries. The conventional interpretation would be that rebellion reflects rejection of official values and of the legitimate means to pursue them (Merton 1968). This interpretation was discussed with groups of respondents. Questions were also asked about the extent to which the new heroin cultures provided a sense of belonging or mutual support, as had been described in the past, or whether any such sources of solidarity had long gone. In the opinion of one new user:

> To tell you the truth I don't feel I am behaving in a rebellious manner. Nor do I feel that I am part of a "culture" or a community of heroin users. I sense that I am different from the others who use the same stuff I use. As far as I am concerned, I just like heroin, and I have a relationship with heroin, not with the others who use it. Some like gambling, some others like big cars or sailing boats, I like heroin. If it were legal and free I wouldn't bother anyone. I have been politically active in the past, but now I am convinced that things cannot be changed within the time I expect to be living. If a better society will ever take shape, this will be when I am not around any more. That's why I want to live well and now.

Along with these straightforward arguments, more nuanced attitudes were recorded among the users that sounded like justifications for both use and dealing:

> In the past I have been politically involved too. I remember one of the slogans that gained momentum in the mid and late 1970s: "death to the distributors of death". We all thought that the dealers were responsible for pushing the youths to drug use. Things have completely changed now. I need my dealer badly and I too could turn into one if required by the circumstances.

Many dealers justify their activity on the basis of being users themselves. They make a point of not being economically motivated. Moreover, they stress how their position entails both the risk connected to use and the "hassle" connected to dealing:

When you use it you don't see anything diabolic in it. Nor do you consider it to be dangerous like you read in the paper. And after all, I also feel reassured that I am doing the right thing. Look around you and see what are the dominant values in this society... I feel entitled to despise such values. Why should one feel "guilty" in a society that thrives on corruption?

Look at all these nice law-abiding people: they do worse things than we do. Think of all the corrupt administrators, the entrepreneurs who illegally traffick arms, the rich who evade taxes. But also think of all the shopkeepers who never give you a receipt so that they can claim a lower income to the tax officers.

These arguments are not simply "techniques of neutralization" (Sykes & Matza 1957). They imply something more, namely an absolution covering everyone, including themselves and those regarded as the "real law violators": those in a position of power. These attitudes imply that everyone, in such a corrupt society, is authorized to behave illegally. Large-scale illegalities are deemed tolerable by the small dealers who then feel that their own "small" illegalities can be condoned. This may be a reflection of broader developments in recent Italian popular culture, which is perhaps getting so accustomed to administrative and entrepreneurial corruption that such corruption is almost expected as a natural characteristic of those who are in power. This acceptance, however, also encompasses self-indulgence and complacency: "I condone the illegalities of the powerful so long as I can engage in my own illegalities as a powerless individual". But are the two types of illegality commensurable?

A key issue, as in other socioeconomic hierarchies or markets, is power: the weak and vulnerable live in the shadow and at the mercy, of the powerful and strong. As users admit:

There is a ruthless hierarchy among us. The more vulnerable, those who need the substance more badly and are unable to hide their need, those who lose control or get sick publicly, are kept at a distance and despised. Those who use the stuff on their own and control the effects, those who use a purer heroin, perhaps because they also sell it, are respected and looked at with admiration.

A paradoxical market, where the more keen the consumers are – the less well they are treated by those who supply the commodity they demand!

The lower the position you occupy in the hierarchy the more you are loathed. The thing is that, as a user, you are regarded as unpredictable; you could do anything, incapable of self-respect, you can be blackmailed by the police. Instead, those who *deal*, use the stuff themselves, and perhaps offer some to their friends from time to time, or those who along with the stuff can even buy their friends a meal and a bottle of good wine, are highly respected. One must learn to act big, to show lucidity and proficiency, be successful in the job and with women.

For most heroin users today, memories of a strong relationship between political activity and heroin use are beginning to fade.

I was very young when I joined the youth section of the Communist Party. I also joined some political groups who were active in the college where I studied. We used to smoke joints and perhaps we didn't take politics very seriously, but at least politics was a way of staying together and doing something collectively. However, heroin was a real taboo. But then . . . disillusionment. Politics didn't bring any immediate results, but at least it gave me the impression that I could complain about the things I didn't like, I felt that I had a right to complain. Today I can't even do that. Now, when I meet other users like me I always hope . . . that we may engage in some sort of discussion. In my circle many have a need to talk, to say their opinion about things, but they never get a chance to do so.

There are still many users who feel a kind of political rather than moral distaste for the idea of buying heroin in order to re-sell it at a profit. The social figure of the "small shop-keeper", the cornerstone of entrepreneurial culture, was one ridiculed by the youth movements of the 1970s, and among the early heroin users, and the image and values conveyed still attract contempt. Moreover, the refusal to deal in heroin resonates with the ideological principle of "refusal of work", which was a part of the radical agenda of left political movements in the 1970s.

> Selling is also stressful, perhaps more so than just scoring. Think of M., who is so generous and so unfit to act as a shop-keeper. He used to give smack on credit to anyone. In this way he would go "in the red" for millions of lire, with the risks and consequences that you can imagine when he had to pay back those who sold the stuff to him. And again, what kind of life is that for the dealer? Appointments at fixed times, always be vigilant, meet the customers, have a walk around together to see if everything is all right, collect the money, go and get the stuff, another appointment on a different street corner, pass the doses, and so on. It is a stress, it would be lethal for a person like me.

Some users aspire to a less mundane lifestyle and a higher standard of living. This is the case with those who were already "skilled" criminals before the growth of the heroin economy and for whom possession of cocaine or heroin became a status symbol, as wealth. This was also the case with some who had become "skilled" as a part of their daily search for money to buy drugs. As one informant confessed: "In the periods when I give up, I find myself penniless; I don't even have money to go to the cinema or to the bar. The absurdity is that, when I use heroin I am stimulated to do anything, for instance I manage to steal more recklessly and daringly than when I am 'sober'. You see, when I use heroin I also have money in my pocket, I can live decently. When I stop for a period I also become broke. So, I do like heroin, but I also like spending money on other things, I also like living well".

As we might suspect, a different ex-user argued that such accounts are probably rare. In his view, the heroin scene and its participants generally tend to be more unassuming and far less daring.

After all, the life-style of many heroin users is closer to that of an ordinary worker. They work all the time; and two or three times a week, instead of going to the cinema or away for the weekend, they have a fix. This is also the case with the habitual users. The scene changed radically, there is now a general decline in standards among those who score and sell heroin. In the past we used to be united, . . . I am convinced that today, when one decides to give up heroin, one does so out of disgust. You give up because you have had enough of the heroin scene, not because you are fed up with heroin.

As for the values shared by the habitual users, an ex-user suggested this interesting parallel:

> Those who use heroin today do not see any specific values that they share with other users. Many perceive themselves as ill. They feel as though they need a blood change from time to time, or as though they have a kidney disease and need a daily renal dialysis. The heroin world is obsessive, it is like living in a hospital, where everybody keeps talking about their illness, and where the only subject of conversation is the common condition of illness.

Not all users see contemporary drug cultures as dominated by competition and lack of friendship, support or solidarity. Heroin users, they argued, are like all social groups and produce relationships, social life and rules: in fact, among heroin addicts, the "dishonest" may be censured more than they would be among "normal" groups.

Looking back over these accounts, it should be acknowledged that at times respondents were somewhat contradictory. Reference by new users to rejection of- or sympathy with – old political movements and principles, might have been employed as part of a repertoire of techniques for self-justification. It is also true that many heroin addicts describe themselves and their lifestyle in terms which draw upon externally produced descriptions offered by popular media and expert commentators. This seems to prove the validity of the principle that a so-called double-hermeneutics operates in sociology and society, whereby the dissemination of interpretations of social phenomena interacts with the actors, who then appropriate and utilize them, thus reproducing or creating new social phenomena (Held & Thompson 1989).

In Turin, heroin use started during a period of high politicization, but despite the decline of political activity it can be argued that it is not legitimate to claim that there is a wholly clear and neat cultural divide between the early politicized heroin users and the current "new" users *(La Repubblica,* 23 February 1990; Arlacchi, Lewis & Turri 1988, Arlacchi & Lewis 1990). In Italy, this argument has been over-used and applied too broadly to the heroin scene of every Italian city be it Naples, Bologna, Verona or Milan. In Turin, politicization was too profound for its traces to be wholly washed away, although not everyone would agree with this view – in particular those who see themselves as the original and unique, politically aware pioneers of heroin use. For them, there is certainly a cultural gulf between themselves and the new users, who lack any such political grounding and who are instrumental in "perpetuating conformity". In interpreting such political and cultural shifts, it is impossible to make definitive statements. We might argue that the former view has some validity for some users, but we leave the last word to the scathing judgement of one ex-user:

> Many users today live like industrial workers: go out in the morning, hustle without knowing who you are working for; buy a substance of which you know nothing, use a substance without knowing why. This is alienation. Once, the use of heroin incorporated some collective rituals: we would inject it together because we wanted to stay together, like in a dinner party. Today, each user has a fix in complete isolation. Today, at the most, heroin users may become business partners, for a moment. They do some business together, but do not share the same culture. After all, many users have no other interest in life than heroin: if you took it away from them, they wouldn't know what to do with their time. This is why the therapeutic communities of a religious kind have a grip on them: because they substitute the void with an allegiance, the nothing with an exaltation, with a new god which will inevitably require their dependence and, ultimately, addiction. The city of Torino, moreover, with its factory discipline, also imposes a par-

167

ticular rhythm on its heroin addicts. Get up early in the morning, go to work, hustle, score, everything to be done at precise times of the day, the times accepted by the productive rhythm of the town. The last shot is at ten in the evening, when the "normal" people watch their last programme on TV. Then everybody to bed, because the following morning one has to get up early, to start all over again.

The market structure and diverse participants

Compared to its counterparts in several other major Italian cities, Turin's heroin market is a secondary one. Two main systems of distribution operate: the first involves members of organized groups based in Milan, and the second draws in autonomous indigenous groups. The latter may comprise both independent mid-range criminal groups who are not (or not yet) recruited by larger organizations, and mixed groups of users and dealers who appoint a courier for one-off operations. Amsterdam remains the most common destination for these amateurish distribution co-operatives, but other overseas sources might be India or Thailand. In the late 1970s, this "autonomous amateur" type of distribution accounted for 30–40 per cent of heroin supply in Turin (Gallo et al. 1980). The remaining supply was provided by "emissaries" of organized crime operating in the region of Lombardia. Turin was therefore a submarket, where a measured deal would normally be 20–30 per cent more expensive than in Milan.

The representative of the distribution group based in Milan, who ended up settling in Turin, supplied mid-range dealers and was personally responsible for the transactions. He would rarely store, or even "see" the drug, as he had people working for him to physically handle the consignments. Until a decade ago, the evaluation of risk involved in these transactions must have been rather favourable because:

> [Transactions involving] consignments of heroin, of quantities between half a kilo and one kilo, occurred once a day. One went to the appointment, showy cars would arrive, el-

egant gilded individuals would come out followed by younger men who were just as elegant and visibly armed. They would take the money but they wouldn't give you the stuff immediately. Instead, directions were given as to how you would get it. A second appointment would be given, a little later, and someone else would hand you the little parcel. Today things are much more complicated: consignments of that quantity only occur once every ten days. This is entirely due to security reasons (dealer).

Despite their high visibility, these early heroin distributors were widely tolerated because of fears that any intensive police response might expose a wide-range of other established, highly profitable illicit activities. In these communities it was inevitable that familiarity with heroin would grow and that it would slowly be incorporated into local illicit economies as a new commodity, with the potential to be more remunerative than anything previously dealt with. As a mid-range distributor describes:

In some areas the local illegal groups were against drug trafficking. Many were afraid that drugs would bring more police into the area and that their business would be disrupted. If you run an illegal betting office or a clandestine gambling business, or buy and sell stolen car parts or other stolen goods, you never call the police in your area, that's for sure. You don't even if you operate at low level, like selling contraband cigarettes.

In time, inevitable police intervention in these areas justified such fears. Long established illicit business activities were closed down or displaced, arrests made and a localized economic "black hole" left in place. Many who were previously hostile to drug dealing, were thus drawn to the drug economy, which did not require a fixed geographical location and hence offered the prospect of anonymity and security.

The heroin market of Turin seems to have maintained the characteristics of a sub-market for most of the 1980s. Middle sized groups have either fought for or agreed with one another over zones of influence. Only one specific period was allegedly marked by the near monopoly of one organization. This was between 1982–4, when the media-labelled "clan of the Catanese" virtually dominated distribution in the town. The power of this group, spearheaded by the Miano family, crumbled in 1984 following various arrests and defections. Generally, the Turin market conforms to a state of loose and unstable oligopoly. The organized crime groups with Milan connections are not the only wholesale operators and a significant dimension of the market is left to other families and groups whose share may vary from time to time. In Turin there is no monopoly of control or activity in the drug economy. As a social worker explained:

> It is wrong to imagine a mega-organization that controls everything. We have to think of different groups which control specific sectors of the heroin market and simultaneously control other illegal activities carried out in those specific sectors. Many dealers, in other words, are also fences and deal with a wide range of goods. Among our clients, for instance, some users pay for their drugs in gold, that they somehow steal, and materially never see money. The money transaction occurs between the dealer and those (traffickers) who provide them with heroin, and it is up to the former to decide how to find money to pay back the latter.

The Turin heroin market is supplied by various routes and sources. Refined heroin arrives from other regions of the Italian Peninsula: Apulia, Campania, Sicily, Veneto, Calabria, and each of the leading groups in Turin relies on its own source of provision. According to a plausible map suggested by the daily paper of Turin, and based on consultation with the "Nucleo Operativo dei Carabinieri", the principal criminal groups in the province of Turin have been: the Sicilian Mafia, three different families of the Calabrian "ndrangheta", a powerful group from Apulia, and an indigenous Piemontese group in alliance with local Gipsies (*La Stampa*, 16 June 1989). In this report a climate of competition was described and evidence was given of alliances between the groups, producing a condition of "unstable oligopoly". The consequences of this fragmentation of the market were perceived by an habitual user as follows:

Firstly, the quality of heroin is getting increasingly worse. At the same time, as the competing groups are growing in number, so are the number of mid-range transactions carried out. This means that the risk of heroin seizures increases as well, with the consequence that the street price of a dose rises. You have to consider that such transactions are more hazardous than importing

For this reason, it was suggested, those who imported directly from abroad could gain access to the market, establish competitive prices and at the same time reduce risk and present a more professional image.

A second consequence of a fragmented market has been the increase in the number of dealers handling medium quantities. This, along with the increase in the number of users, resulted in more cuts to the drugs being dealt. In turn, the decline of quality was viewed as a signal that a growing number of inexperienced people who were just looking for an income were entering the heroin market. The dealers interviewed described some suppliers as non-users, connected to large scale organizations, with the capacity to handle sums averaging 2 billion lire (£1 million), and weights of heroin up to 5 kilos. They also estimated that a dozen mid-range distributors deal with quantities of heroin around 1 kilo. A smaller dealer who obtained his supply from one of the latter argued:

> If these mid-range distributors were blocked, the entire market would collapse. True, it is very difficult to identify those who supply heroin to them, but if the intermediaries were caught, there would be no heroin at all on the market . . . when one of these mid-range distributors is arrested then suddenly we don't find smack. All the hype that heroin is everywhere is only hype. When the supply is blocked you don't know which way to turn.

It was suggested that these 1 kilo level distributors could earn up to 10 million lire a day (£5000), though lower level dealers wanted to make a point of stressing how "ordinary" their own earnings were: "I buy between 50 and 150 grams each time. In terms of money I handle 10 million lire each go. If I wanted I could earn 10 million lire a day. But I don't feel like it, I am under too much stress. I am scared, and I only keep my long-term customers, those who can't cope without me".

At the next level down, the dealers interviewed estimated there were between 30 and 40 people handling quantities of heroin below one kilo and above a hundred grams. Around one thousand people were estimated to be handling quantities measured in grams. The former passed the substance over to a fixed number of the latter, who were their stable customers. As one dealer put it:

> There is a lot of heroin around. The problem is how to sell it. Over the last few years many people have entered the heroin business and now the market is literally overcrowded. You see, the reason for this is that it is very easy to find someone who invests money in heroin, it is also easy to find those who are prepared to sell it; what is difficult is to raise the demand at the level of supply. I am not talking from the point of view of the users, who always have to keep in touch with the heroin scene if they don't want to be left without. I am talking of small and medium transactions. When I go and buy 100 grams, for example, I am always told to buy a kilo instead, because it would be cheaper and I am also told not to worry: payment will be discussed another time.

Competition and fragmentation in the market, along with the entry into distribution of new dealers who know little about the drugs they sell, not only makes for commercial uncertainties but may also have fatal consequences for users. For example:

> Someone decides to enter the market; all they do is throw a large quantity of heroin into the market at low price. The quality of the dose is no longer checked: it's chaos. When there is abundance of heroin, the demand for small dealers consequently increases, because more retailers are needed to sell all that stuff. So, in some areas of town, you see fourteen-year-old boys handling a number of doses. For them it's work, in a market that suddenly is in bad need of labour. The new employees are inexperienced, don't know how to cut the doses, and consequently risks for the users soar. In

this activity people don't have time to gain experience, nor to learn skills. One may have been a grocer one day and suddenly the next, instead of selling salami he finds himself selling heroin.

The introduction of North African street dealers into heroin distribution has been described in a similar way. Previous experience of cannabis dealing was not sufficient preparation for a shift to dealing 40 to 50 grams of heroin, a substance that these dealers were unfamiliar with, either chemically or commercially. An Italian daily newspaper described these new dealers as "manual workers exploited by criminal firms", dealing in the courtyards of their own homes without adopting the minimal precautions that even rudimentary experience would prompt (*La Stampa*, 28 March 1990).

What became of the more independent, autonomous networks of distribution that, in the early 1970s, provided 30–40 per cent of the heroin used in Turin? First, the consortium model of distribution was limited to small-scale transactions and pretty much disappeared. In part this was because it could not offer producers a steady demand and hence negotiate favourable prices. In addition, larger importers frequently reported these amateurs, their unlikely competitors, to the border police. The possibility of engaging in independent trafficking can, therefore, seem increasingly remote, especially for those not wise enough to make peace and preliminary agreements with those groups controlling local distribution. Sooner or later, most of the "independents" have been forced to enlist themselves as "dependents" of larger and better organized groups. This is the status quo. However, not everyone is satisfied with its constraints.

The courier's story

The following account is from a dealer who tried to shift from dependent to independent work. In this description, the dynamics at work between informal consortia and organized groups emerge as more complex than the simple distinction between "mafia trafficking" and "hippie trafficking" would suggest.

I was arrested with 300 grams of Thai heroin. I had another 200 grams concealed in my rectum. I had been an independent courier before, because I didn't want to work for any organization any longer. A trip to Thailand only makes sense if a quantity of at least 300 grams is bought. Travelling expenses have to be accounted for, along with the stay and with the costs in terms of risk. You see, many people are prepared to pay as much as 7–800,000 lire [£400] for a gram of Thai. I am talking about 85% pure substance, excellent stuff that can only be found where it is produced. Once the stuff has reached Italy, it can even be retailed: you just sell a few grams to those you know. Or you sell the bulk to someone who will then cut it and resell it to small distributors. In this way, the journey would bring me the value of at least 100 grams, and in my case, an habitual user, problems were resolved for a good while. Obviously I gave a very pure substance to the distributor, one that absolutely had to be cut before being put on the market. Otherwise the casualties would have been numberless. So I had to be very careful as to who I was dealing with: it had to be someone I trusted, who knew their job. I know, one of these journeys should be enough to settle down economically for ever. But I was only interested in smack for my own use and, at the same time, I was keen to travel for the sake of it.

. . . My being arrested left me a bit suspicious. The fact is that they already knew I was passing the frontier. I have no idea whether they were tipped off by someone in Thailand, or someone from Italy. They probably knew already about me when I left Italy, but they let me go first and then stopped me on my way back. I sensed anyway that at the border they were sure I had heroin on me. They showed unexpected tenacity and self confidence. The dogs didn't signal a thing, and yet the police insisted, they were certain. I thought that my name had been given to them by the organization for which I'd worked before. The fact that I had gone independent may have caused jealousy.

Until 1988, this informant had worked for an organized group and was paid 10 million lire each trip (£5000). The operations he participated in were not explained to him in their entirety and he was only briefed on one task at a time. Large organizations act in this way for security reasons and to allow for the unpredictability of indecisive couriers who may change their mind about what they are being asked to do. This informant continued:

> I still wonder how could they trust people who were so rootless or simply desperate? Perhaps they were confident of their own power and the terror they could instil. They played on their punitive capacity, including the possibility of just dumping you, for instance by reporting you to the police.

Sometimes even finding a way to conceal the drugs was left entirely up to the courier. Typically, he said, he would only be told the first airport where he would land, and that once there he would be given a new ticket to his next destination. Once back in Italy, even after delivering the smuggled drugs, he was not paid immediately. Instead he says, he had to "pursue, almost beg" the person with whom he was in contact. When he was paid, he was "ripped off" with only a part of the money due being paid in cash, the remaining part being paid in heroin. This was unfair, because the quantity of heroin he received was valued in terms of the street level price – not the price at which he had bought it in the producer country. He continued:

> Next trip everything would change again. The contact person was different, the stop-overs were different and the whole operation would be structured differently. True, once you know the distributors who operate abroad you can try and go independent. But you need finance, and once you take the stuff to your own town you must know the distributors or the users and dealers you can sell to.

An attempt to move into independent trafficking can evidently be attractive and rational where past experience has been dominated by exploitation, lack of protection and insufficient support. Funds to cover travel expenses did not take account of this smuggler's need for heroin for personal use: "heroin users are regarded as scum, tramps who don't deserve any respect". During the journey back to Italy he was generally followed by a member of the organization who did not make himself known. "I didn't know who this passenger was, he was flying with me, he could have been one of those dressed like businessmen. In such circumstances you can't try to be clever: if you think you can disappear with the stuff you are mad".

The successful courier can come to occupy an impossible (and unenviable) position in coming to be regarded as so proficient that fears develop that he will double-cross the organization and seek to become self-employed.

> When I went independent, I could do a good job with something like 10 million lire [£5000]. I could collect money from a number of people I knew and who would be interested in the business. These people were users who would also sell small quantities. Four or five trustworthy people like that can take turns in making the trip and set up a little autonomous firm. Moreover, in these cases, if you are arrested, at least someone will take care of you, sending money to prison and paying for a good barrister. Sure, autonomous trafficking is also very dangerous, but at least you are respected within your circle. I took personal risk, and on top of that I was also a user. Nobody in my circle of friends could say that I was an opportunist. The others who contributed money would not take any risk, so I had to take care of the whole operation, and provide the stuff for everybody. For this reason I was admired and respected: I was seen as brave and honest. Nobody could dare say that I had an easy life or that I exploited others. The situation was ideal, both for me and for my friends. But I'm sure this type of thing may have annoyed someone, and when it became common knowledge that we were operating in this way, someone decided that intervention was necessary.

This takes us back to the beginning of the courier's story.

The overlap between the legal and illegal economies in Turin

So far we have sketched the rôle played in the heroin market by ex-robbers, organized or independent groups. We will now examine the involvement of individuals who are not part of the conventional criminal underworld.

In Turin, the corruption of the legal economy by illegal elements has taken place alongside two other major processes which have characterized the recent history of the town. These are the processes of industrial decentralization and that of neo-liberalization (Ruggiero & Vass 1992). A vast literature is available concerning industrial decentralization (Amin 1989, Bagnasco 1988, Deaglio 1985, Paci 1982, Trigilia 1986). In Italy, this process induced an "economic miracle" by developing a parallel economy where statutory requirements are frequently ignored. Small production units were established employing fewer staff than traditional workshops, which meant that trade union agreements need not apply. Overt illegalities are committed in many of these units with respect to working conditions, wages, security, recruitment etc. In this model of production, chains of such small units and workshops are often set up by a parent factory for cost-saving purposes (Del Monte & Raffa 1977). It is in this network of ancillary production, where the boundaries between legality and illegality are already blurred, that shifts towards criminal activities often occur (Ruggiero 1987).

Among the sub-contractors who produce components for the parent industry, various types of "nuovel entrepreneur" take their chance. Some are directly appointed by the big firms, which may entrust loyal employees with the running of a small ancillary firm. Some others, who compete with the large firms, have "adventurous", if not criminal, backgrounds. Among these, some are simply re-investing the proceeds of criminal activities in legal productive activities. This world of small industries is animated by cross sub-contracts, privileged alliances, mutual favours and joint ventures of all types. In this hectic network of negotiation and business, many "clean" entrepreneurs may undergo the opposite process to that undergone by their ex-criminal colleagues. In other words their interests may occasionally move from the legal into the illegal economy.

One dealer described an approach from such investors:

> I have been approached by people who had no relationship with the heroin scene. Business was proposed to me. . . . In a place like Turin, small entrepreneurs, traders or profes-

sionals are within the circle of people somehow connected to someone who uses heroin. Well, some of these traders and professionals proposed themselves as investors. They didn't want to know in what their money would be invested, or perhaps they just pretended not to know. I have done these operations with them a few times, especially when I had difficulties in paying back my supplier.

In other circumstances, it may be the dealers who seek money for investment in their business:

It was I who proposed the business. I did so to the owner of a mechanic workshop I knew. He had never used any drugs, but he had acquaintants in the drug scene. I asked him for some money, and I assured him that I would pay back the sum with 40% interest. He understood, and the operation was concluded. Some other traders or small entrepreneurs would start by saying that they had financial difficulties or that they were poised to launch a new activity . . . then would come up with a proposal.

Examples of such cases have involved estate agents in the town and proprietors of night clubs. The latter may not have accumulated money by means of illegal activities, but:

they were "clean" people who slowly came into contact with a largely criminal set of customers: smugglers, robbers, and so on. After a while, they just sell their connivance, as they tolerate all wheeling and dealing going on under their nose. They sometimes become partners in some business with their own customers. They can also act as "money-lenders" or "money-launderers", they can sell information, provide a hiding place, and the lot. It is as if they "rent out" their private premises and their clubs to the heroin distributors. It is obvious that in such places you can find anything: guns, cannabis, cocaine and heroin.

Along with small entrepreneurs and others in business, it is also possible for the unemployed to seek a solution to financial problems in the heroin economy. Some may carry out a single operation, with the aim of starting a self-managed business in the legal economy. Thus:

> Some people just plan to earn a certain amount of money and then give up. They try their chance in one go, then set up some clean business. A friend of mine did something like that: he was a courier for once only, then he did another deal like buying and reselling 200 grams of heroin. He now runs a "pizzeria" on the Spanish coast.

The ideological (re-)emphasis placed upon market forces in western economies may also have played an important part in stimulating areas of overlap between legal and criminal activities. Earlier we termed this process neo-liberalization. In Turin, neither the cultures of accommodation and negotiation nor a formalized "market mentality" have been particularly strong. An abrupt neo-liberal triumph within a society that is already largely deregulated therefore ends up by eroding further the already uncertain boundaries between legal and illegal behaviour.

One recent example of "clean" entrepreneurs getting involved in criminal activities and being subsequently sentenced, hit the headlines in 1990. These businessmen were sentenced for kidnapping and heroin trafficking (the proceeds of the former being invested in the latter). In court, one of them remarked:

> I am an entrepreneur, and before committing those offences I had to deal with the ferocious financial world. This world is dominated by hypocrisy and throat-cutting competition. I had to resolve my economic problems, pay the wages to my employees. As for the persons we kidnapped, we thought: it is better to inflict pain in one go and only to one person, than to damage innumerable people in the daily struggle to survive . . . Each time we would say to ourselves it was the last, but then we would do it again. Our firms were going bankrupt, and fresh money was constantly needed (*La Stampa*, 6 May 1990).

Other legal firms have limited their rôle to money-laundering, processing the criminal proceeds entrusted to them by dealers and traffickers through their banks and retaining a percentage as commission. Another recent case centred on a group of "clean" Piemontese financiers who were recycling funds derived from the local heroin business and from a sensational robbery carried out, some 800 km away, in Rome. In effect, for some time they were acting as a nationally renowned centre for money-laundering, a position which they gained by virtue of long-term experience as well as by operating in an allegedly Sicilian mafia-ridden area of the country.

Some other legal entrepreneurs act as unofficial loan providers and are known in the underworld of Turin as "prestasoldi" (money-lenders). Usually they have no criminal record and prefer to bargain with mediators who, in turn, have access both to criminal and to legal firms. The money-lenders enjoy the confidence of their banks and easily get loans which they pass on to the mediators, who then return the sum, adding an agreed interest percentage.

From the "professional" criminal to the "mass" criminal?

In the Turin criminal labour market, and the heroin economy in particular, we suggest that the present picture is one of relatively few professional criminals at the apex and an increasingly large sector of petty offenders at its base. These petty offenders do not possess any particular skills, face a limited degree of career mobility, and will usually be expected to perform only routine and repetitive tasks. Those arrested for possession with intent to supply, in fact, represent a relatively constant quota of users, interchangeable, frequently arrested and easily replaced.

Many addicts arrested are unknown to detoxification centres or the police. It is therefore likely that they are mostly neophytes in crime. As we have noted above, a recent Italian phenomenon is that many new users finance their habit through their legal income, while trying to keep their heroin use compatible with a conformist lifestyle. Those who do commit offences, repeatedly engage in crimes which offer relatively little financial reward.

These observations were discussed with users and dealers, who compared them with their own experience and reflections. In general, there was agreement about the picture presented but respondents were keen to put matters in perspective. Many started by emphasizing the significance of the distinctions between the various levels constituting the distribution hierarchy, thereby emphasizing their own importance or unimportance. But one key factor was consistently noted, at the top and in the middle positions, *professionality* is crucial, and it was felt that this is often acquired during time served in prison.

Prisons and the process of professionalization

One of the dealers interviewed claimed that he had been approached in "Le Nuove Prison" of Turin by a large distributor who had heard of his previous activities and reliability. The dealer claimed that he had, in fact, been hoping for just such an approach which could offer him an introduction to a more professional and organized range of contacts. His reasoning was that when the "route to Amsterdam" was interrupted, the only real suppliers were to be found among organizations operating in Milan and their representatives in Turin, hence "getting on" in the drugs business required breaking into a higher level in the hierarchy. In Lombardia (the region of Milan), heroin laboratories had been set up which have only recently been discovered by the police (*La Repubblica*, 23 May 1990, 24 May 1990). To do business on a larger scale, one had to either to go Lombardia or work with those bringing heroin from there to Turin. For this dealer, it proved unnecessary to travel to Lombardia and try to make contacts; the prison system facilitated this for him. A different long-term dealer recalled his own realization that the times and the market were changing: "We, the more vulnerable, had all fallen. We were so naïve: we thought we could travel freely and continuously without raising suspicion. I kept going and coming from Amsterdam and I didn't realize that my time had come. Once in prison, it became imperative for me to contact those who had taken over and were now controlling the distribution in town".

There is no doubt about the professionality of this informant. He had already acquired skills during a history of long-term criminality but now, as a result of his prison contacts, he is developing them further. The dealers who serve time in prison sense that their future is decided there, a future which depends on how they negotiate the experience and the contacts they make there. A dealer argued:

> In prison I never thought I would give up. Once released, I planned to do things better. I met people who advised me as to where I could find the same stuff at a cheaper price. Someone said I was crazy travelling abroad: I could get a better deal in Italy, around the corner. In prison everybody knows everything about you: who you are, what you have done and above all how you have behaved with the police and in court. If you are identified as a suitable person, they come along and propose business. In sum, if you are arrested with, say, two grams of heroin, when you get out you'll have much more than that. You learn a lot inside, you develop good connections. If you are trusted you get a more steady position when you get out.

In a similar account, a contrast with the past was highlighted:

> In the past you could meet brave and trustworthy people in prison. Projects could be planned with these people, and partnerships set up once you got out. Prisons were like examining boards, where the more serious and lucid would be promoted, and those who panic would fail. Today you don't look for business partners any longer. The best contacts you can make are with large organisations which can give you a job. They are not partners though, they are your bosses.

During the Turin research, varying degrees of professionalism were described, a finding which does not enable us to generalize or draw neat distinctions. Some individuals combine typical professional characteristics with the more limited skills and ambitions of the category we have termed the "mass" criminal. This was the case, for example, with small-scale dealers who handle quantities of heroin up to around 10 grams. They are required to have some expert knowledge of the drug, and of the techniques to package, conceal, and sell it. On the other hand, such activity is routine, repetitive and far from specialized. Furthermore, such individuals are replaceable, precariously insecure and often paid on commission. Some couriers are in a similar situation, especially those who feel exploited in spite of the real skills they have acquired during the course of a long and risky learning process. These skills, as described earlier and in the following account, frequently receive poor acknowledgement or reward from employers:

> As a courier I was paid on commission, but I didn't find it satisfactory. It happened like this: I already had a reputation as a serious guy. I used to sell little quantities in order to have my own supply for free. I was regarded as reliable, cool, I paid my debts regularly. You see, this is one of the most important problems for the organisations: how to find someone who is reliable and willing to work for them. But on the other hand, the courier is entrusted with too many tasks and is required to have too many qualities: he must be emotionless, be professional in hiding the stuff; he mustn't crave a hit, never use the stuff while working. A good courier might know the drug well because he uses it, but he must also have a detached relationship with the substance, otherwise he would be unable to work. You need a professional. But would a professional accept such work as a courier?.

Unsuccessful couriers may (willingly or unwillingly) slide back to the position of street dealers. In Turin, even the head of the police department recently lamented the decline of criminal professionalism in the town and the stability and standards that had been associated with it. With the increase of what he called "microcriminality", the tasks and expertise of the police are being stretched to the point where they feel disorientated:

> Increasingly, our units must work in close conjunction. Our field of action is forced to widen. Until a few years ago, armed robberies, for example, were exclusively undertaken by professional gangs. Today you never know who it may be: it may be very inexperienced guys, heroin addicts, all sorts of crooks. Our expertise must encompass property crime, drug addiction, and other connected things (*La Stampa*, 18 May 1990).

In the same vein, the head of the prison service in Turin expressed profound disenchantment. Perceptively he argued that prisons are becoming like the "general hospitals" of past centuries as they increasingly hold individuals who are not serious criminals but "sick" people who need doctors, psychologists and social workers. As elsewhere in the west, the idea of imprisonment as providing custody and rehabilitation for serious criminal offenders is giving way to a rôle for prisons as warehouses for problem populations or as high security hospitals for those who would be better served by proper medical care.

As one user observed:

> Prison does not boost everybody's career. Some may fall even lower and become completely subdued, enslaved. I mean subdued by the system but also enslaved by heroin. In every institution it is very easy to find drugs, and most prisoners don't object to them. This is understandable: drugs are the main topic of conversation in prison. Today, the majority of inmates are behind bars because they have done something connected with drugs; those who have a lot of money have made their money with drugs; those who are desperate have become desperate because of drugs. Those who have never tried heroin end up by using it as soon as they have a chance.

The heroin economic cycle: use, distribution and crime

The heroin economic cycle resembles other industrial cycles, where commodities, production and distribution can be relatively independent of consumption, use and effects. Some respondents suggested that even mid-range distributors do not "know" much about heroin. They are neither aware of the cycle of production nor are they very clear about why the commodity is sold and bought. If the notion of "professional" should include an understanding of the overall productive process (i.e. the transformation of raw material, the finishing of a product, etc.) then we must conclude that in the heroin economic cycle in Turin, true "professional work" is rare – even given the impetus to professionalization which rising levels of imprisonment have promoted.

Street sellers and users are kept in low level service rôles by the bigger distributors and, as a consequence, a self-labelling process builds on assumptions of inadequacy and the acceptance of low expectations. One drug worker elaborated on this mix of self-labelling and structural determination:

It is curious how many heroin users never make the leap into dealing. They don't even when they have a desperate need for the substance and dealing could resolve their problems quickly. The thing is that users who are in bad need cannot hide their condition, so that nobody would trust them for any business. On the other hand they also reach the conviction that they are unreliable, that they are good for nothing. They may claim that they don't want to deal because they haven't got a shopkeeper's mentality, but in actual fact they feel incapable, inadequate. Others feel useless because they come from a working-class family. To them work is waged work, it is dependent work. For this reason they would find it hard to go independent; at most they get a dependent job in a criminal organisation, but they'll never become small entrepreneurs. To them dealing heroin would be like running a business.

The daily routine for this class of unskilled labour entails situations such as the following:

There is a general atmosphere of despair. The risk of being arrested is so high that the repercussions are felt in every moment of the day. It is getting increasingly difficult both to find money and to get hold of smack. Let me give you an example. If you have permanent contacts with the heroin circle, one day the word goes around that you can score on that street corner at seven o'clock in the morning. The dealer won't wait. There, a second appointment is set up for the sake of security: eleven o'clock on another street corner. This is a sort of flying dealing, and it is very stressing, agonising. Some don't make it, some can't cope with such rhythm, but they are forced to go on. (social worker)

Scoring is not the only hectic activity in which habitual users are involved. The following accounts describe other aspects of this life under constant pressure. This is a daily routine of repetitive tasks performed in a segmented economic cycle over which little or no control can be exerted. "Mass" criminals are tied to the assembly line as rigidly as Fordism has bound other workers. Here for example, are some rather unexciting job descriptions:

We have to discover new places all the time. Turin is a burnt territory: the town has already been ransacked. Shop assistants are suspicious. A lot depends on how you are dressed. It also depends on self-control. But sometimes I am fidgety, excited, so I can't do a thing. Every day the target must be chosen carefully, or even better a list of targets must be prepared, just in case things don't go well. Sometimes it takes a whole week to get some money. Then when you get some you can relax for a short time.

The truth is that even when you have some money you can never stop worrying. Money and drugs run out quickly, and so while you are injecting you already think about the next time you have to find money to inject again. This is my life, I am always on the ball, also because I am only able to do good jobs when I have used the stuff. If I don't fix I become incapable of stealing.

Burglaries are very difficult. Very few of us are able to do them: you need to be cool and expert. You also need a lot of patience: know where you're going, and prepare the thing properly. We don't have that time and ability. We only shoplift, amid infinite difficulties. Generally we are neither together enough to burgle a house nor desperate enough to do those muggings that the papers describe as "syringe-armed robberies".

After the theft the stress is not over. It is exhausting to negotiate with the fence. If I bring him a video without a remote control, he immediately plays on this, and says that the video is worth half the price. He knows very well that in shops TVs and videos are displayed without a remote control, but he takes advantage of the situation. I think he has someone who specializes in stealing remote controls, so he plays the same game on two fronts.

Then of course sooner or later we are arrested. It is always the same scene. The police may start beating us up, and we have learned that the only way to stop them is shouting that we are HIV positive. You should see them: their arm stops mid-air. When arrested, I immediately claim I am an heroin addict. I do so because I want to be taken to the hospital where I get methadone. And in prison, the same scene again: the psychologist, the doctor and others, always the same people.

Here, at the bottom of the Turin drug market hierarchy are the poorest users, the petty criminals – the "mass" criminals. They are seen as the lowest of the low and attract the contempt not only of wider society but also of others in the drugs economy. According to a social worker who has visited heroin addicts in prison nearly every day for years:

Something has changed in people's attitudes. Years ago, petty criminals, smugglers, but also armed robbers, were looked at with a subtle form of respect. In some circles they were regarded as honourable criminals, endowed with a strong personality and, after all, as freedom lovers, brave and adventurous. Heroin users are now regarded as weak, losers, slaves both of the drug and of a boss who dictates to them. Heroin users are seen as more disquieting individuals than the traditional figures involved in crime. Their condition is seen as the result of "vice", "weakness", from which they are unable to escape: they are loathed because of their lack of self-control. Moreover, heroin users make illegal choices which do not bring any visible advantage in terms of status: and for this reason they are all the more scorned.

Ironically, in Turin, as elsewhere, the heroin economic cycle actually benefits (directly or indirectly) a large proportion of the population. Stolen goods find many customers in town, fences set up agreements with users with a view to accelerating the circulation of goods, and specific orders for particular goods are made and met.

Paradoxically, users persist in individualistic, competitive street and petty crime which benefits them little and is very risky, while servicing an economic sub-system that could provide far higher rewards if they were organized co-operatively. But the days of such political thinking are gone: market *individualism* prevails. As a result, bizarre versions of the work ethic take shape. In the words of one long-term heroin user who has absorbed the entrepreneurial spirit of the 1980s and 1990s:

> I may be part of an elite because I am a very skilled thief. Some are real wrecks and lack the imagination and the energy to do what I do. But, many just don't want to understand that they have to take their situation seriously, as if they had a real job. They have to dress properly, go out in the morning and find the way of getting hold of some money. My point is: Do you like smack? Well, don't harm anybody, don't mug an old lady, don't cheat a friend and don't rip off people like you, who need the same stuff as you do. Get up in the morning, shave, get dressed and go to work like everybody else. You see, some are lazy, and prefer the humiliation of asking others. Sure, I am talking about the weak ones, the real wrecks, and I am sure that this kind of person is found in any job or profession. But many are not just unable to do anything, they are bloody lazy.

A psychologist with 10 years experience of working with heroin users, suggested a profile of "mass" criminals based on their high rate of activity but low degree of control over, or inclination to understand, the heroin economic cycle in which they are caught:

> Many lack any motivation, they can't spell out or identify the reasons underlying their choices. If you ask some youths who live in the peripheral zones of Turin why they use heroin, they don't know what to say. It is like asking them why they watch TV. They use heroin because it is there, it is part of the scene. They don't even grasp how heroin is by now part of the local economy in which they themselves play a very important rôle. If heroin disappeared, whole urban areas would economically collapse.

Have you ever wondered why the shop keepers of the periphery are so wealthy? This should make us suspicious if you realize that in those areas the unemployment rate is very high and the official average income very low. Heroin produced wealth; even the small legal economy, in some parts of the town, is buttressed by the drug economy, thanks to the work of an army of desperate youths.

Conclusion

This chapter has described aspects of the development of the heroin market in Turin and of the political and social background, characteristics of heroin users, dealers and large scale distributors, and the phases through which cultures and ideologies of heroin use have moved. Importantly, we hope we have also illustrated how the modern prison is more of a stimulus to the professionalization of drug-crime than reform and rehabilitation. Finally, the chapter has contrasted the significance of such professionalism with the emergence of a new and growing, unskilled/de-skilled, criminal underclass, the "mass" criminal.

Here, as in earlier chapters, we have sought to draw attention to parallels with and connections between the legitimate/licit market economy, the grey area of semi-legal activity, and the growth, diversity and significance of the illegal/illicit drug economy. Current debates in sociological theory concerning features of late-modern society and Fordist/Post-fordist models of production, may suggest ways to develop our analysis of the particularities of this Italian case study, or our London study, further. Our conclusion draws together themes and conclusions already presented and discusses the validity of our initial hypotheses in the light of the material presented.

6

Conclusion: comparative remarks

In this concluding chapter, we shall consider aspects of the relationship between the illicit drugs economy and the legal economy and discuss the validity or invalidity of the hypothetical propositions we outlined in Chapter 1.

Illicit and licit economies

Our examination of the relationship between the drug economy and the legal economy in Italy and England, and in particular in the cities of Turin and London, suggested that there are certain key differences which are worth emphasizing.

In Turin, the connections between criminal and legal enterprises seem to have reached the sphere of what is called "industrial productive capital" and we have described the way in which some small legally-productive firms, born out of industrial decentralization, have become involved in criminal activities. These legitimate firms are central to modern systems of industrial production in Italy, yet many are to be found among those "clean" companies which are heavily or peripherally engaged in the drug business and other criminal activities. Convergent interests are found in these decentralized units, where, on the one hand, criminal groups may invest the illegal proceeds of crime, and on the other, adventurous entrepreneurs form alliances with their illegal counterparts in search of (untaxed) profit levels that are difficult, if not impossible, to achieve through legal enterprise.

In London, the legality/illegality overlap can be found principally in the economic sphere where import and export companies and general "commodity traders" operate. These companies may take advantage of established, legitimate commercial links with countries that produce illegal drugs, in order to camouflage their illicit drug importation (Ruggiero & Vass 1992). Alternatively, such business interests may use a legitimate "front" to conceal large to medium scale distribution activities, or related money-laundering. Examples of the latter include car and van hire firms and dealerships, restaurants, amusement arcades, nightclubs, art and antiques dealers, florists, and bureaux de change (Dorn & South 1990, Dorn et al. 1992b on "sideliners"). In classical economic terms, this encounter between reputedly "clean" business and illicit drug activity in London, seems to take place in the domain of "commercial capital".

In London, the essential elements that seem to have favoured the success of drug importation enterprises appear to have been: the accessibility of sources of production, the existence of legal communication channels with these sources, and the ability to mesh legal commercial operations with illicit trafficking. Distribution enterprises also take advantage of the latter facility as well as the availability of the resources necessary to underwrite large financial transactions and the physical disposal of large quantities of an illegal commodity. The variable availability of these resources may explain the variable degree of involvement of the different London ethnic groups in trafficking. These groups rely on their specific legal channels of communication, which usually coincide with the routes leading to their respective country or region of origin. The variety of drugs imported is therefore *partly* dependent on where importers can establish legal commercial links. On the other hand, of course, much smuggling simply attempts to circumvent all legal channels and avoid over-reliance on overseas partners or suppliers. The former relationship of dependence, probably figures most where connections based on family and ethnic ties are involved; the latter, a relationship of suspicion, is more characteristic of the xenophobic mistrust of "foreigners" exhibited by traditional, white "criminal diversifiers". Production and distribution of synthetic drugs such as MDMA (ecstasy) or LSD, imported for example, from the Netherlands, will require less reliance on ethnic or family connections and may rely more on purely commercial (e.g. traditional criminal or legitimate investors), "fraternal" (e.g. Hells Angels) or "ideological" (e.g. rave culture) motives and understandings. In Britain, insular concerns about the opening of European borders may, therefore, have some limited foundation but also be in need of serious re-thinking (Dorn 1993b, 1994). First, the British drug market has strong relationships with drug producing (e.g. in Asia) or key transit (e.g. in the Caribbean) countries that, by and large, correspond to the countries of its ex-empire and former spheres of influence. Secondly, there is some evidence that, while some drugs arrive in Britain from European countries such as Holland or Spain, others follow the reverse route, from Britain to other European countries. For example, the first ecstasy dealers ever arrested in Italy were white British nationals, as were a group of crack distributors recently arrested in Paris.

The white "criminal diversifier" groups operating in the London market are usually well structured, with well established influence and interests in local illicit markets where other illegal commodities have traditionally circulated (cf. Hobbs 1988). Their proven ability to move a wide variety of stolen goods and illegal items has placed them in an excellent position to carry out drug distribution effectively. For some, success in developing distribution has served as an incentive to attempt to develop import operations as well. In this way, profits are maximized, as control is extended across the cycle from production to sale – from international trafficking to home distribution. However, we might note that a strong presence in the London drug trade is no guarantee of success in attempts to emulate 19th century colonialist capitalism. Both dealers and police reported that white importers had been "stung" and, like legitimate international enterprises as well as international drugs enforcement agencies, have found that having credibility and power in London, Rome, Washington or wherever, may count for little when negotiating in Afghanistan or Colombia.

Five hypothetical propositions about European drug markets

Returning to our initial hypothetical propositions, outlined in Chapter 1, we shall consider their validity and invalidity in the light of our discussion so far.

Hypothesis 1

The first hypothesis seems to be validated: the explosion of drug availability, in both the case study contexts, has contributed to and stimulated an increase in organized forms of drug-related crime. In particular, this has occurred in the higher reaches of the distribution hierarchy. However, this tendency can perhaps be attributed less to demand for drugs *per se* than to the illegality of the market in which they are sold. As many commentators favouring decriminalization or legalization of drugs have argued, the escalation of organized forms of crime can be interpreted as the inevitable outcome of the parallel escalation of the war against drugs (South 1995a). The increasing efficiency of state drug enforcement agencies may have contributed to the trend towards more structured operations taking place in the drugs economy (Dorn & South 1990). Drug distributing firms and enforcement agencies should be regarded as interacting. The impulse towards a greater degree of criminal organization at higher levels of the drug economy can be seen, therefore, as the consequence of such interaction, rather than an endogenous process "naturally" accompanying the evolution of illicit markets. We have noticed this occurring in both the case study contexts described. The nature and direction of innovation in drug-crime enterprises are also the consequence of specific repressive policies which rely on certain types of intervention. Dorn & South (1990) offer a similar analysis of how certain developments on the enforcement side, in particular covert operations and surveillance of cash-flow,

> press hardest against those distributors with larger and relatively static organisations, resulting in a market inhabited by a range of small, loose and flexible organisations. Other developments, in particular the long term cultivation of informants and a repeated escalation of penalties, have pushed the trade in the direction of becoming more security conscious, more prepared to use violence to deter informant and enforcement agents, and in general more brutal: the trading environment has been shaped in ways that attract high risk-takers (Dorn & South 1990: 78).

Hypothesis 2

The second proposition to be tested was the popular view that drug markets and trafficking are dominated and/or controlled by monopolies or large cartels – with Mr Big directing all. As we had expected, this proposition was largely invalidated by our research findings. In reality, this view over-estimates the capacity of a single organization to control the market and dominate each segment of it within the over-used model of a pyramidal structure. In addition, it places excessive emphasis on tendencies towards monopoly which, in fact, tend to lose out in the conflict with counter-tendencies of a competitive nature (cf. Reuter 1984). In effect, in *both* contexts studied, we found a situation where a number of competing distribution enterprises coexist, and where monopolistic tendencies gain momentum only periodically. Only for a brief period of time did Turin witness a situation of virtual monopoly, its more familiar profile being characterized by the co-presence of mid-range groups which operate on a local and circumscribed level. This distributive model was also observed in London, where small and middle-range firms operate and only periodically engage in territorial competition.

Drug distribution is carried out by diverse and changing groups, a circumstance which leaves space for erratic and amateurish ventures. In London, attempts to monopolize the market may be frustrated by various factors and forces, not least the market variable of consumer power or choice. When monopolies are tentatively established, and consequently prices increase, users' demand may shift to other products or cocktails, be they legally or illegally obtainable. Furthermore, the very urban and social geography of the city makes London less a homogeneous metropolis than a cluster of socially and ethnically diverse villages. In this situation, even if monopolies in the distribution of drugs can be established within one area or "village", economic, ethnic, cultural and even logistical differences will prevent the extension of monopoly across other parts of the city.

Hypothesis 3

In the third of our hypotheses we speculated on a shift from what we have termed "crime in association" to "crime in organization", a shift which we believe is favoured by the growth of drug-crime enterprise. We defined the former model as implying a horizontal structure, characterized by individual and group entrepreneuriality in a non-hierarchical market. In the terms of classical sociology, the division of labour here is "technical". "Crime in organization" on the other hand, is characterized by a vertical structure; its industrial and corporate style of conducting business implies the exchange of "criminal labour" for payment (in money or drugs) – a wage relationship is created. The "McDonaldization" of drug enterprise suggests what we mean here and it is described at its most elaborate in the work of Johnson et al. (1985) on the division of labour found in New York heroin markets. In classical terms, this division of labour is of a social nature.

As regards Italy, the involvement of organized crime in the importation, distribution, and on some occasions the production of drugs, is by now extensively documented by both judicial evidence and sociological research findings. Moreover, it is acknowledged that these activities acted as a powerful incentive for traditional criminal organizations such as the mafia to step up involvement in legal large-scale business. The proceeds of the drug business have simply been too large to be entirely channelled back into the drug industry or other illegal economies. This hypothesis certainly seems valid for the case study of Turin, where the shift from "crime in association" to "crime in organization" was confirmed in the accounts of many respondents. However, both imported drugs and drugs refined in Italian laboratories are sold to wholesale distributors who do not necessarily belong to traditional criminal groups or families. These middle-range distributors have never been "men of honour" in the traditional sense of mafia membership, but were previously involved in professional criminal activities which they conducted in an independent fashion. Among them for example, are armed robbers whose involvement in the drug business resulted in the loss of their previous autonomy. Small-scale distributors, user-distributors and finally pure users certainly epitomize "crime in organization" as they are employed in a structure where planning and execution are strictly separated.

However, we have found that to attempt to apply the concept of "crime in organization" in relation to Britain, and in particular to our London case study, meets with some deeply rooted difficulties.

Our hypothetical definition of "crime in organization" was partly coined in an effort to avoid the usual problems posed by the term "organized crime" when applied in the British context. Here, a customary assumption is that this term is principally associated with the Italian-American model of criminal groups. We believe that these groups only represent one variant of "crime in organization", whereas our attempt to provide an alternative term encompasses other elements and variants found in Britain and other European countries.

Some traditional traits still characterize "crime in organization" in Italy, though these coexist with new forms of business orientation and entrepreneuriality. These traits are mainly related to the huge muscle- and fire-power of traditionally structured groups, which in a sense can rely on a true "army". Quasi-military force is still a crucial feature of the variant of "crime in organization" prevailing in Italy. This is not the case with the organizations operating in London, where the use of firearms is certainly increasing but, by comparison with Italy or the USA is far less frequent and by no means always associated with drug-crime. Our informants in South London, for example, remarked that the use of firearms in their area has usually *preceded* the involvement of criminal groups in the drug economy. Armed robberies, for example, may be carried out to generate the preliminary accumulation of funds, which may then, or eventually, be invested in a drugs deal. In other words, the use of firearms is certainly a disturbing reality in the British context but it is not an element which *distinguishes* the form of "crime in organization" prevalent in British cities (Ruggiero 1993a). It is noticeable, however, that media reports and enforcement interests may gain something from emphasizing links between arms and drugs, whether this is substantiated or not.

It has always been possible to sell one's "criminal labour power" in exchange for a wage, and the expansion of the alternative illegal economies, in large part stimulated by the growth of drug trafficking and distribution, has correspondingly expanded criminal opportunity structures. Hence, one way of trying to make sense of the drug distribution structures set up in Britain is to apply industrial models (although this should not be taken to imply a heightened degree of "professionalism"). The crime "industry" (cf. Mack & Kernes 1975), like any other industry, requires a workforce of senior and middle management and, of course, a large number of unskilled criminal employees. It is the necessity, presence and contribution of these employees that should be regarded as a significant hallmark of "crime in organization".

The development of the drug business in both Turin and London has been accompanied by shifts away from independent activity and small-scale, locally networking groups, towards a market that is increasingly dominated by many competing but more organized firms. This is not a shift to monopoly control nor have all the small and independent operators disappeared – it is highly unlikely that they ever will. But increasingly, the market involves straight-forward economic relationships, the manipulation of "wage-dependence" as well as drug dependence, and hierarchical divisions of labour and authority. In Britain, some features of the structure of the drug business do appear to be close to our definition of "crime in organization". These are: the possibility of selling one's criminal labour in exchange for a "wage", the applicability of an industrial model to the illegal activities connected to drug distribution, a corresponding work hierarchy and a segmentation of rôles, a blurring of normative boundaries between acceptable and unacceptable productive activities, and, relatedly, the partial overlap of the legal, semi-legal and the illegal labour markets.

Examples of crime that could be described as "organized", "syndicated" or "crime in organization" have been the subject of surprisingly few studies in British criminology (see Hobbs 1994). One possible explanation for this is that British examples generally lack the sensational or sinister characteristics which have been held to characterize the familiar American forms of "traditional" organized crime (Clarke 1990). In the 1990s however, there are clear indications that much has changed since Mack first wrote of "the Crime Industry" in 1964. British crime enterprises may not appear to resemble the Italian–American variant of crime in organization: a clandestine, highly professionalized "army" of the type familiar in Sicily and Italy is redundant in the type of "firms" operating in British cities. However, the sheer scale of the profits and developments that have arisen from the growth of the drug economy in Britain, Italy and throughout Europe, might suggest that in the future, British criminal enterprises are likely to become more organized and more visible than in the past. At some point in the future the lack of mafia-style "soldiers" may indicate only a quantitative rather than a qualitative difference between the two variants.

As Campbell (1990: 8) observes:

> In a way, what has happened to British crime parallels what has happened to British industry. The old family firms . . . have been replaced by multinationals of uncertain ownership, branches throughout the world, profits dispersed through myriad outlets. . . . The 1990s is seen as a boom time for them, with the exploitation of a recreational western culture that wants its luxuries and its drugs. The legitimate business will run alongside the illegitimate ones.

Hypothesis 4

We have suggested that the growth of the drug market has provided a major boost to the broader illicit economy and also led to the traditional "professional criminal" being increasingly overshadowed by the "mass" criminal. This suggestion needs further assessment. The material we have gathered and examined suggests that, as we might expect, an increase in unskilled crime does not automatically result in criminal professionality as a whole becoming redundant. In Turin and the north of Italy, we found both mass criminals and professional criminals involved in the drug economy. Perhaps unsurprisingly, many ex-armed robbers have simply refined and transferred their skills. In some cases, therefore, a rise of professionality in the drug business was observed in the Italian case study. A similar process seems to have taken place in London and here too, professional crime has re-skilled, re-developed and diversified into non-traditional areas of activity which offer high profit potential – drugs, fraud, etc.

De-skilling, the "industrial model" and crime

As well as similarities, there are of course profound differences between drug markets in Italy and England and one explanatory factor is a technical but simple one. The average purity of drug deals sold in Turin and in other Italian cities may be as low as 1–3 per cent, whereas "bags" sold in London have reached about 30 per cent purity (Wagstaff & Maynard 1988). This may suggest that, in the Italian context, the drug economy employs a far higher number of individuals and groups, each taking their "cut" within a more intensively stratified structure. This also suggests a different degree of "massification" in the two contexts examined. Many more individuals are attracted to the drug economy in Italian cities than in Britain (Lewis 1989). In this respect, the situation in many Italian cities seems to be closer to that of North American cities, where the drug economy encourages a range of related activities, individuals with diverse skills are recruited, and where drugs generate the circulation of money and goods that underpins a broader parallel, non-drug economy.

In terms of general trends, the decline of criminal professionality in some activities seems to have been accompanied by the rise of professionality in others. Activities such as "fencing" – which can be a large-scale activity far removed from the old-time small, "pawn-shop-type" fence – are a classic example of criminal enterprise stimulated by the drug economy. Here, inexperienced labour is "managed" by those with access to distribution networks for stolen goods (e.g. high performance cars). The process of deskilling at the bottom of the new crime hierarchy fosters new managerial skills at the top.

The steady growth of unskilled acquisitive crime may have further repercussions, fostering the spread of other antisocial behaviours which are damaging to daily life in inner-city communities. In other words, activities connected to the drug economy may make a significant contribution to the so-called "broken window" effect. This occurs in a situation of urban decay characterized by diffuse antisocial behaviours: housing policies which label certain estates and neighbourhoods as "dumping grounds"; the loss of services and shops and the evaporation of credit and insurance cover (Wilson & Kelling 1982, Hope & Shaw 1988). The creation of such areas has proved crucial for the spread of drugs in both the contexts examined.

In the Turin case study, we have noted the tolerance with which the first drug distributors were greeted by traditional criminal groups and participants in the irregular economy. This tolerance is understandable in terms of the desire of such groups, who were not involved in the drug business, to keep the attention of the authorities away. In time, some of these groups did move into the drug business. We also noted how some individuals, who had no previous involvement in crime, turned to the drug business after familiarization with established distributors. In the London case study, we have suggested that racism and the "otherness" of the black population makes even a remunerative criminal career a problematic option. A similar phenomenon can be observed in many Italian and other European cities, where the characteristics of the "mass" criminal increasingly appear to be fulfilled by the "visible" immigrants operating in the drug economy. In Turin, for example, North Africans are commonly employed as low-level wage-earners in the criminal economy. This has been accompanied by their subordination, low professionality, high vulnerability, and lack of knowledge regarding the drug economy or the goods they sell.

Hypothesis 5

Late modernity and the influence of Anomie and subculture theories
In this final section, let us move from empirical and analytical matters to theory. Here we shall consider the value of the principal sociological theories traditionally employed in analysis of drug use – subculture theory and the "retreatist" category within Anomie theory (Raymond 1975) and explore our proposal that they deserve re-appraisal.

Merton's reworking of Anomie theory explains deviant behaviour as the result of an incongruity between socially shared goals and the available means to achieve them (Merton 1968). His celebrated typologies, defined as "deviant adaptations", take different forms "depending on the nature of the antinomy between the goals dictated by the dominant culture and the ways in which they are pursued" (Ponti 1980: 261). Merton postulates different forms of adaptation to this conflict including the category of *retreatist* behaviour. Retreatists are defined as those who give up on both the official goals and the means to achieve them. They are conventionally seen as voluntary societal dropouts or involuntary failures, unable to cope with the demands of everyday life. Groups such as alcoholics, vagrants, tramps and drug users are usually cited and are held to be in society but not part of it.

In Cloward & Ohlin's (1961) elaboration of Merton's theory, a distinction is made between: a stable criminal subculture, a conflict subculture, and again a retreatist subculture. The first describes full-time criminals who seek income through illegal means. The second pertains to individuals who are not particularly economically motivated, but who will employ violence to achieve status among their peers. The third subculture encompasses those who experience a "double failure": they are unable to achieve status through either legitimate or illegitimate means. One way of resolving their "status dilemma" is to retreat into the world of drugs. This approach synthesises and elaborates upon anomie theories on the one hand and subculture theories on the other. The classic exposition of the latter is A. K. Cohen's (1955) work which adopted a "social learning" approach and suggested that deviant behaviours are internally transmitted within a social subgroup where these behaviours are already routinely adopted.

These theories are still widely referred to in analysis of the cultural values and motivations of drug users and dealers. This occurs despite challenges to the notion that the social worlds of drug users are characterized by passivity and retreatism (Pearson 1987b). Instead there is a substantial amount of research showing that the variables such as status, success, career, activity, etc. (however limited they may be) are crucial for the understanding of both drug users and distributors (Finestone 1957, Sutter 1966, Feldman 1968, Hughes et al. 1971, Hughes 1977). Such research may be ignored because it presents an image that is difficult to accept in a society where all deviant behaviours are regarded as abnormal or inexplicable. We have already mentioned the pioneering study by Preble & Casey, and here it is worth quoting from their classic article "Taking care of business":

Heroin use today by lower-class, primarily minority group, persons does not provide for them a euphoric escape from the psychological and social problems which derive from ghetto life. On the contrary, it provides a motivation and rationale for the pursuit of a meaningful life.... If they can be said to be addicted, it is not so much to heroin as to the entire career of a heroin user. The heroin user is, in a way, like the compulsively hardworking business executive whose ostensible goal is the acquisition of money, but whose real satisfaction is in meeting the inordinate challenge he creates for himself (Preble & Casey 1969: 21).

The original and supporting material reported and reviewed in this book in relation to Europe, is consistent with Preble & Casey's findings in New York, and their description of the daily routine of heroin users might also be applied in the case of other illicit drugs. Among respondents in our case studies, retreatist behaviours and escapist attitudes were fairly hard to find among either users or distributors.

Anomie and subculture theories deserve re-thinking and critique not only because they fail to account for the recent development of drug use and distribution but also because of other limitations, regarding race, gender, labour market participation and so on (Dorn & South 1988, McRobbie 1980). Their applicability to the changed and changing nature of criminal activity in advanced societies at the end of the twentieth century, could also be questioned. Anomie theories carry the weight of ideological assumptions that reflect their "Americanization", not least the belief that adherence to official goals and means can be widely generalized. Anomie, in fact, offers a plausible interpretation of deviance only if the cultural goal of success is seen as monodimensional, and the drive towards conventional success also prevails among those who lack opportunities to achieve it (Box 1983). Merton's cultural goals refer to a system of norms and values which are regarded as unitary in society. However, late-modern, post-industrial societies are characterized by a plurality of cultural goals that vary according to individuals and the position their social groups occupy. In effect, it is no longer clear that all members of disadvantaged groups share and aspire to conventional goals and/or the means to achieve them. Critical criminology has long argued that among the less privileged, the achievement of these goals seems unrealistic, entailing a drastic limitation of ambitions and prompting a search for more viable strategies for social reproduction (Taylor et al. 1973).

A similar observation has been made by those critics who see Merton's analysis as a surreptitious attempt to make the goals of one dominant part of society relevant to society as a whole. His cultural goals are allegedly derived from a universal human patrimony but in fact only reflect the lifestyle of middle-class America, to whose values all other classes are expected to conform (Gouldner 1970). Aspects of Merton's theory may, therefore, perhaps be more valid when applied to the explanation of white collar and corporate crime (Box 1983, 1987).

The debate related to Mertonian concepts and the examination of the critical literature devoted to them would require a separate essay. It would be necessary, for instance, to revisit the contributions of labelling theorists, symbolic interactionists, ethnomethodologists, conflict theorists and so on. Similarly, a critical assessment of subculture theories and the objections now addressed to them, might occupy the space of an entire book. The idea of "subculture" remains powerful and useful of course. Whatever its limitations it will remain a key sociological concept – even though, as Gallino (1978: 704) argues, its use may often be inappropriate:

> a subculture can be identified only if the elements we observe in it are systemic in nature; only when its composition, structure, and the regularity of events recurring within it form a distinctive sub-system as opposed to the official system, rather than presenting with an indeterminate stack of elements more or less haphazardly coexisting.

Drug use and distribution involves social groups which are too diverse for them to be identified with one or more specific subcultures. It is characterized by extremely mobile subgroups, whose members may shift between different socioeconomic contexts, none of which provides an exclusive source of identity for them. Indeed, the static image that the idea of "subculture" implies seems increasingly less applicable and relevant to youth trends in late- or post-modern society (Redhead 1993). Subculture theories are also excessively indebted to aetiological explanations of crime and deviance which rely heavily on poverty and disadvantaged social conditions (Ruggiero 1993c). To reject such explanations would be foolish but at the same time, of course, it cannot be argued that deprivation accounts for all drug-related behaviour. The activities of many users, dealers and traffickers do not always constitute "forms of adaptation" to a reality which denies them legitimate goals and the means to achieve them. Nor can they always be interpreted as acts aimed at redressing the balance of one's disadvantaged social condition. Within the case study contexts we have examined, it seems increasingly hard to find widespread conscious or unconscious identification with a *distinctive* subculture, especially if we define a subculture as "a system of values which upturns the shared set of values in the respectable and law-abiding society" (Baratta 1982: 75). Polydrug use, heterogeneity of cultural styles, commercialization, depoliticization – all figure in the late modern drug scene (although old characteristics like racism and sexism carry on as ever).

Justifying accounts in drug markets

We have already noted that individuals operating in the drug market may "displace guilt" onto other groups and individuals that they consider more powerful though not less dishonest – an account of particular significance and justification in the context of our Italian case study. Broadly speaking, this type of self-justification can probably be found at every level of the drug distribution hierarchy, whereby all feel that higher illegalities or immoralities are found among those who occupy a higher position in it than they themselves do. In a sense, displacement of guilt proceeds as if in an infinite chain. This is reminiscent of some categories of accounts elaborated by Sykes & Matza (1957) for their explanation of the process of "drifting into crime". Techniques of neutralization, they argued, allow people to rationalize their behaviour and justify themselves and their deviant acts while roughly adhering to the official social norms – or saying that they do. One can read the diffuse "conformism" of many involved in the drug scene in similar terms. Among the techniques of neutralization most frequently invoked in our interviews were the self-assuring claims that Sykes & Matza designated as: the denial of responsibility, the denial of the existence of the victim, and the condemnation of the condemners (Sykes & Matza 1957). However, these categories, which were originally coined to interpret the crimes of the powerless, seem today to apply also to the crimes of the powerful: the "non-existence of a victim" and the "condemnation of the condemners" are put forward even by those at the top of the drug economy (and increasingly, also by those "legitimate" entrepreneurs who break the rules and are caught out by regulatory bodies). Each individual involved in the drug business may easily point to examples of corporate crimes that are or should be deemed more serious and damaging than their own offences. The legitimate entrepreneurs of Turin who invest in the drugs economy, provide typical examples of how even corporate criminals may employ such neutralization techniques, justifying their involvement in drug trafficking and kidnapping, by displacing guilt and cause onto the "ruthless financial world" in which they participate. In all manner of ways, the drug economy cannot be understood without reference to the formal, legal economy.

Finally, let us consider our own sins. In observing the behaviour of others, we may frequently assign attitudes and other characteristics to them that they do not actually have, but which arise out of the expectations of the observers – what Boudon (1989) calls the "projection of dispositions". No doubt in this book we have been as guilty of this as most. We hope, however, that we have at least provided a useful and original account and that others may now take the study of drug use and markets in Europe further.

Bibliography

ACMD (Advisory Council on the Misuse of Drugs) 1988. *AIDS and drug misuse, part 1*. London: HMSO.

ACMD 1989. *AIDS and drug misuse, part 2*. London: HMSO.

Adler, P. 1985. *Wheeling and dealing: an ethnography of an upper-level drug dealing and smuggling community.* NewYork: Columbia University Press.

Agar, M. 1973. *Ripping and running: a formal ethnography of urban heroin addiction.* NewYork: Seminar Press.

Albrecht, H-J. 1989. Drug policy in the Federal Republic of Germany. See Albrecht & van Kalmthout (1989), 175–94.

Albrecht, H-J. & A. van Kalmthout (eds) 1989a. *Drug policies in Western Europe.* Frieburg: Max Planck Institute for Foreign and International Penal Law.

——1989b. European perspectives on drug policies. See Albrecht & van Kalmthout (1989), 425–73.

Alvarez, F. & M. C. Del Rio 1991. Drug abuse in Spain: epidemiology, policy and health structure. In *Drug addiction and AIDS*, N. Loimer, R. Schmid, A. Pringer (eds), 70–79.Vienna: Springer.

Amin, A. 1989. Flexible specialisation and small firms in Italy: myths and realities. *Antipode* **21**, 1, 13–34.

Anderson, M. 1989. *Policing the world: Interpol and the politics of international police co-operation.* Oxford: Clarendon Press.

Arlacchi, P. 1983. *La mafia imprenditrice.* Bologna: Il Mulino.

——1992a. In Italia crescono i consumatori. *Nuova Polizia* **2**, 8–10.

——1992b. *Gli uomini del disonore.* Milano: Mondadori.

Arlacchi, P. & R. Lewis 1989. Sociologia della droga: il caso diVerona. *Micromega* **4**, 59–98.

——1990. *Dossier droga: l'eroina a Bologna.* Bologna: Regione Emilia Romagna.

Arlacchi, P., R. Lewis, R. Turri 1988. *Il mercato della droga a Crotone.* Crotone: Regione Calabria.

Arnao, G. 1975. Information in etiology of drug abuse in Italy. *Bulletin of the International Council on Alcohol and Addiction* **1**.

Ashton, M. 1986a. Doctors at war – part one. *Druglink* **1**, 1, 13–15.

——1986b. Doctors at war – part two. *Druglink* **1**, 2, 14–16.

Assessorato alla Sanita' 1980. *Relazione sulle tossicodipendenze.* Torino: Regione Piemonte.

Assignment 1993. *Assignment.* BBCTV programme on prospects for legalisation; reporter, Edward Stourton, London, Tuesday, 5 October.

Auld, J. 1981. *Marijuana use and social control.* London: Academic Press.

Auld, J., N. Dorn, N. South 1984. Heroin now: bringing it all back home. *Youth and Policy* **9**, 1–7.

——1986. Irregular work, irregular pleasures: heroin in the 1980s. In *Confronting Crime*, R. Matthews & J. Young (eds), 166–87. London: Sage.

Avico. U. et al. 1990. The impact of new regulations on drug abuse in Italy. In *Epidemiological Trends in Drug Abuse*, Community Epidemiology Work Group. Rockville, Maryland, USA: Department of Health and Human Services.

Baanders, A. 1989. *De Hollandse aanpak, opvoedingscultuur, drugsgebruik en het Nederlands ovberheidsbeleid.* Assen: Van Gorcum.

Bagguley, P. & K. Mann 1992. Idle, thieving bastards: scholarly representations of the "underclass". *Work, Employment and Society* **6**, 113–26.

Bagnasco, A. 1986. *Torino: un profilo sociologico.* Torino: Einaudi.

——1988. *La costruzione sociale del mercato.* Bologna: Il Mulino.

Bandini, T. & U. Gatti 1987. *Delinquenza minorile: Analisi di un processo di stigmatizzazione ed esclusione.* Milano: Giuffre'.

Baratta, A. 1982. *Criminologia critica e critica del diritto penale.* Bologna: Il Mulino.

Barrio Anta, G. 1991. The spread of cocaine in Europe. See Bruno (1991), 144–9.

Baudrillard, J. 1979. *De la seduction.* Paris: Editions Galilée.

Bean, P. 1974. *Drugs and social control.* Oxford: Martin Robertson.

——1991. Policing the medical profession: the use of Tribunals. See Whynes & Bean (1991), 60–70.

——(ed.) 1993. *Cocaine and crack.* London: Macmillan.

Bean, P. & Y. Pearson 1992. Cocaine and crack in Nottingham 1989/90 and 1991/92. In *Crack and cocaine in England and Wales*, J. Mott (ed.), 20–32. Home Office Research and Planning Unit Paper 70. London: HMSO.

Becker, H. 1963. *Outsiders: studies in the sociology of deviance.* New York: Free Press.

——1967. History, culture and subjective experience: an exploration of the social bases of drug-induced experiences. *Journal of Health and Social Behaviour* **8**: 163–76.

Berridge, V. 1978. War conditions and narcotics control: the passing of Defence of the Realm Act Regulation 40B. *Journal of Social Policy* **7**, 285–304.

——1979. Morality and medical science: concepts of narcotic addiction in Britain, 1820–1926. *Annals of Science* **36**, 67–85.

Berridge, V. & G. Edwards 1981. *Opium and the people: opiate use in nineteenth century England.* London: Allen Lane. 2nd edn 1987. New Haven: Yale University Press.

Bewley, T. & H. Ghodse 1983. Unacceptable face of private practice: prescription of controlled drugs to addicts. *British Medical Journal* **286**, 15 October.

Bianchi, M. 1986. *Oziosi e vagabondi: disoccupazione, crisi giovanile e piccola malavita.* Milano: Silvana.

Bieleman, B. & C. Kaplan 1992. Cocaine: widespread but not harmless. *Interna-*

tional Journal on Drug Policy **3**, 4, 187–9.

Bienkowska, E. 1991. Crime in eastern Europe. In *Crime in Europe*, F. Heidensohn & M. Farrell (eds), 43–54.

Bild, M. & P. Hayes 1992. Women drug users and diversion from custody – a view from the probation service. In *Women, HIV, drugs: criminal justice issues*, N. Dorn, B. James, M. Lee (eds), 52–60. London: ISDD.

Blackwell, J. 1983. Drifting, controlling and overcoming: opiate users who avoid becoming chronically dependent. *Journal of Drug Issues* **13**, 2, 219–35.

Blumir, G. 1973. *Con la scusa della droga*. Rimini: Guaraldi.

Blumir, G., C. Caraccia, G. Martinotti 1975. Drugs and the Italian society. Paper presented at International Conference on Drugs and Society, Milan, 15 March.

Bockma, H. 1992. Distributing heroin to addicts is pointless (interview with J. P. Grund). *International Journal on Drug Policy* **3**, 4 193–4.

Bohlen, C. 1993. Russia mobsters grow more violent and pervasive. *New York Times*, 16 August, A1/A6.

Bolton, K. & A. Walling. 1993. User to user. *Druglink* **8**, 4, 14–15.

Bonino, R. 1982. Il caso dei tossicodipendenti. In *Le frontiere della citta': casi di marginalita 'e servizi sociali*, F. Barbano (ed.). Milano: Franco Angeli.

Boseley, S. 1993. A fatal fix of freedom. *The Guardian*, Europe section, 9 March, 14.

Boudon, R. 1989. Razionalita' soggettiva e disposizioni. In *Il soggetto dell'azione*, L. Sciolla & L. Ricolfi (eds). Milano: Franco Angeli.

Bourgois, P. 1989. In search of Horatio Alger: culture and ideology in the crack economy. *Contemporary Drug Problems* Winter, 619–49.

Boutmans, E. 1989. The situation in Belgium. See Albrecht & van Kalmthout (1989), pp. 89–106.

Box, S. 1983. *Power, crime and mystification*. London: Tavistock.

——1987. *Recession, crime and punishment*. London: Macmillan.

Brecher, E. M. 1972. *Licit and illicit drugs*. Boston-Toronto: Little Brown.

Bruno, F. (ed.) 1991. *Cocaine today: its effects on the individual and society*. Rome: UNICRI (United Nations Interregional Crime and Justice Research Institute).

Bruun, K., L. Pan, I. Rexed 1975. *The gentlemen's club: international control of drugs and alcohol*. Chicago: University of Chicago Press.

Buchanan, J., S. Collett, P. McMullan 1991. Challenging practice or challenging women? Female offenders and illicit drug use. *Probation Journal* **38**, 2, 56–62.

Buning, E. 1992. Harm reduction in mainstream thinking. *International Journal on Drug Policy* **3**, 4, 182–5.

Burr, A. 1983a. The Piccadilly drug scene. *British Journal of Addiction* **78**, 1, 5–19.

——1983b. Increased sale of opiates on the black market in the Piccadilly area. *British Medical Journal* **287**, 883–5.

——1984. The illicit non-pharmaceutical heroin market and drug scene in Kensington Market. *British Journal of Addiction* **79**, 337–43.

——1987. Chasing the dragon: heroin misuse, delinquency and crime in the context of South London culture. *British Journal of Criminology* **27**, 4, 333–57.

Butler, S. & M. Woods 1992. Drugs, HIV and Ireland: responses to women in Dublin. In *AIDS: Women, Drugs and Social Care*. N. Dorn, S. Henderson & N. South (eds), 51–69. London: Falmer Press.

Caballero, F. 1989. *Droit de la drogue*, Paris: Editions Dalloz.

Campbell, D. 1990. *That was business, this is personal: the changing face of professional crime*. London: Secker & Warburg.

——1993. Police seize heroin in tomato lorry. *The Guardian*, 20 November, 1.

Cancrini, L., M. Malagodi Togliatti, G. P. Meucci 1977. *Droga: chi, come, perche' e soprattutto che fare*. Firenze: Sansoni.

Carter, B. & M. Green 1995. Naming difference: "race thinking", politics and social research. In *The social construction of social policy*, C. Samson & N. South (eds). London: Macmillan.

Catanzaro, R. 1988. *Il delitto come impresa: Storia sociale della mafia*. Padova: Liviana.

Censis (Centro Studi Interventi Sociali) 1986. *Ricerca sulla mappa di diffusione del fenomeno della tossicodipendenza e sulla quantita' e qualita' degli interventi pubblici e privati in Italia*. Roma: Ministero degli Interni.

Chambliss, W. 1977. Markets, profits, labor and smack. *Contemporary Crises* 1, 1, 53–76.

Chambliss, W. & R. Siedman 1971. *Law, order and power*. Reading, MA: Addison-Wesley.

Chatterjee, S. 1989. The limitations of the international drug conventions. See Albrecht & van Kalmthout (1989), 7–20.

Chinnici, R. & S. Mannino 1983. La mafia oggi e la sua collocazione nel piu' vasto fenomeno della criminalita' organizzata. In *Riflessioni ed esperienze sul fenomeno mafioso*, Consiglio Superiore della Magistratura (eds). Roma: Arti Grafiche Jasillo.

Christie, N. 1989. Reflections on drugs. See Albrecht & van Kalmthout (1989), 41–8.

Chrusciel, T. 1990. Drug services in Poland – yesterday and tomorrow. In *The years ahead*, P. Fleming (ed.), 10–22. Winchester: Wessex Regional Health Authority.

Clark, D. 1980. Smack in the capital. *Time Out* 51.

Clark, V. 1993. Murder is boss as mob rule comes to fairy-tale city. *The Observer*, 8 August.

Clarke, M. 1990. Syndicated crime in Britain. *Contemporary Crises* 4, 403–420.

Cloward, R. & L. Ohlin 1961. *Delinquency and opportunity: a theory of delinquent gangs*. London: Routledge & Kegan Paul.

Cohen, A. K. 1955. *Delinquent boys: the culture of the gang*. New York: The Free Press.

Cohen, P. 1989. *Cocaine use in Amsterdam in non-deviant subcultures*. Amsterdam: Instituut voor Sociale Geografie.

Cohen, S. 1972. *Folk devils and moral panics: the creation of the mods and rockers*. London: MacGibbon & Kee.

Coluccia, A. 1990. *Norma giudirica e tossicodipendenza in Francia*. Milano: Giuffré.

Commission of the European Communities 1990. *Report on the national programmes to reduce the demand for drugs in the European community*. Brussels: CEC.

Community Epidemiology Work Group 1986. *Community epidemiology work group proceedings, June 1986, Volume 2, selected issues: AIDS, drug abuse and crime, ethnographic research, international research*, Rockville, MA: NIDA.

Cooney, P. 1991. *Report drawn up by the Committee of Enquiry into the spread of organized crime linked to drugs trafficking in the member states of the European Community*. Luxembourg: Office for Official Publications.

Corrigan, D. 1979. The identification of drugs of abuse in the Republic of Ireland during the years 1968–78. *Bulletin on Narcotics* 31, 2, 57–60.

——1986. Drug abuse in the Republic of Ireland: an overview. *Bulletin on Narcotics* **38**, 1/2, 91–7.

Cotic, D. 1991. A comparative overview of legal drug control. See Bruno (1991) 204–6.

Courtwright, D. 1993. Should we legalize drugs? No. *American Heritage* February/ March, **43**, 50–56.

Customs and Excise 1983. *Annual drug seizures*. London: HMSO.

——1990. *Annual drug seizures*. London: HMSO.

Dally, A. 1983. Drug addicts in Piccadilly. *British Medical Journal* **287**, 22 October.

——1990. *A doctor's story*. London: Macmillan.

Dahrendorf, R. 1987. The erosion of citizenship. *New Statesman*, 12 June, 12–15.

Daniel, P. 1993. Problem drug use reported by services in Greater London. In *Drug misuse in Britain 1992*, ISDD/M. Ashton (eds), 69–79.

D'Avanzo, G. 1992. Alle corde i re della droga. *La Republica*, 29 September.

Davies, G. 1992. The cocaine trail leads to eastern Europe. *The Observer*, 15 November.

Davis, M. 1992. *City of quartz*. New York: Vintage Books.

DEA (Drug Enforcement Administration) 1982. Cocaine trafficking trends in Europe. *Drug Enforcement*, Fall, 21–2.

Deaglio, M. 1985. *Economia sommersa e analisi economica*. Milano: Giappichelli.

Dean, A. 1991. Cocaine and crime in Britain: an emerging perspective. See Bruno (1991) 246–53.

Dean, A., A. Carvell, A. Green, H. Pickering, G. Stimson 1992. Cocaine and crack use in Britain in 1990. In *Crack and cocaine in England and Wales*, J. Mott (ed.), 12–19. Home Office Research and Planning Unit Paper 70. London: HMSO.

Dean, G., J. Bradshaw, P. Lavelle 1983. *Drug misuse in Ireland 1982–83*. Dublin: Medico-Social Research Board.

Dean, G. et al. 1984a. *Characteristics of heroin and non-heroin users in a north central Dublin area 1984*. Dublin: Medico-Social Research Board.

Dean, G., R. Smith, B. Power 1984b. *Heroin use in a Dun Laoghaire borough area 1983–84*. Dublin: Medico-Social Research Board.

de Celis, B. 1989. France's policy concerning illegal drug users. See Albrecht & van Kalmthout (1989), 143–60.

de Celis, B. 1992. *Fallait-il creer un delit d'usage illicite de stupefiantes?* Paris: CESDIP.

De Kort, M. & D. Korf 1992. The development of drug trade and drug control in the Netherlands: a historical perspective. *Crime, Law and Social Change* **17**, 123–44.

de la Cuesta, J. 1989. The present Spanish drug criminal policy. See Albrecht & van Kalmthout (1989), 293–320.

Del Monte, A. & M. Raffa 1977. *Tecnologia e decentramento produttivo*. Torino: Rosenberg & Sellier.

D'Este, R. 1990. *Intorno al drago: lo spettacolo sociale della droga*. Torino: Nautilus.

Dianin, G., E. Duckworth, M. Lipsedge 1991. *A preliminary survey of Italian intravenous heroin users in London*. London: South East Thames Regional Health Authority.

Dias, C. & F. Polvora 1983. Drug addiction among adolescents, *Bulletin on Narcotics* **35**, 3, 81–8.

Diez-Ripolles, J. 1989a. Principles of a new drug policy in Western Europe from a

Spanish point of view. See Albrecht & van Kalmthout (1989), 321–42.

Diez-Ripolles, J. 1989b. Current trends on the works of the European Parliament with regard to narcotic drugs. See Albrecht & van Kalmthout (1989), 21–8.

di Gennaro, G. 1982. *La droga*. Milano: Giuffré.

——1991. *La guerra della droga*. Milano: Mondadori.

Ditton, J. et al. 1991. Scottish cocaine users: wealthy snorters or delinquent smokers? *Drug and Alcohol Dependence* **28**, 269–76.

Ditton, J. & K. Speirits 1981. *The rapid increase in heroin addiction in Glasgow during 1981*, Background Paper 2, Glasgow: Department of Sociology, University of Glasgow.

Ditton, J. & A. Taylor 1987. *Scotland drugs resource book: 1980–1984*. Glasgow: Criminology Research Unit, Glasgow University.

Dorn, N. 1993a. Subsidiarity, police co-operation and drug enforcement: some structures of policy making in the EC. *European Journal on Criminal Policy and Research*, 1/2, 30–47.

——1993b. Drug trafficking and enforcement counter measures in Europe: a comparative perspective on public perceptions and policy priorities. Paper to Centre for the Study of Public Order, Conference, Leicester, September.

——1993c. A European analysis of drug enforcement. Paper to European Scientific and Technical Seminar on Strategies and Policies to Combat Drugs, European University Institute, Florence, Italy, December.

——1994. Drug enforcement within Europe: police co-operation in the age of free movement for EC nationals. In *The drugs trade*. London: Howard League for Penal Reform & Bellew Press.

Dorn, N., S. Henderson, N. South (eds) 1992a. *AIDS: women, drugs and social care*. London: Falmer Press.

Dorn, N., K. Murji, N. South 1992b. *Traffickers: drug markets and law enforcement*. London: Routledge.

Dorn, N. & N. South 1984. Drugs and xenophobia. *Marxism Today* **28**, 3, 3–4.

——(eds) 1987. *A land fit for heroin?: drug policies, prevention and practice*. London: Macmillan.

——1988. Of males, markets and sexuality: a critical review of youth culture theory. Centre for Criminology Paper 4. Middlesex University, London.

——1990. Drug markets and law enforcement. *British Journal of Criminology* **30**, 2, 171–88.

——1991a. Drugs, crime and law enforcement: some issues for Europe. In *Crime in Europe*, F. Heidensohn & M. Farrell (eds), 72–83. London: Routledge.

——1991b. Communications, education, drugs and HIV. In *AIDS and drug misuse*, J. Strang & G. Stimson (eds), 162–73. London: Routledge.

——1993. After Mr Bennett and Mr Bush: US foreign policy and the prospects for drug control. In *Global crime connections*, F. Pearce & M. Woodiwiss (eds), 72–90. London: Macmillan.

——1994. The power behind practice: drug control and harm minimization in inter-agency and criminal law contexts. See Strang & Gossop (1994), 292–310.

Downes, D. 1977. The drug addict as a folk devil. In *Drugs and politics*, P. Rock (ed.), 89–97. New Brunswick, NJ: Transaction.

Doyle, L. 1994. Drugs intelligence unit sweeps into action. *Independent*, 3 March, 9.

BIBLIOGRAPHY

Druglink 1991. Heroin haul supports EC border controls. *Druglink* **6**, 2, 6.
——1993. Harm minimisation review planned by Department of Health. *Druglink* **8**, 3–5.
Edwards, G. (ed.) 1978. *Problems of drug abuse in Britain*. Cambridge: Cambridge Institute of Criminology.
Ehrenberg, A. 1992. *Drogues, politique et societé*. Paris: Editions le Monde/Decartes.
Einstadter, W. J. 1969. The social organization of armed robbery. *Social Problems* **17**, 1, 64–83.
Eisner, M. 1993. Policies towards open drug scenes and street crime. *European Journal on Criminal Policy and Research* **1**, 2, 61–75.
Elliott, A. 1992. Drugs and crime. Criminology course journal, Department of Sociology, University of Essex, unpublished.
Engelsman, E. 1989. Drug policy and the management of drug related problems. *British Journal of Addictions* **84**, 211–18.
Enzensberger, H.M. 1977. *Politica e gangsterismo*. Roma: Savelli.
Ettorre, B. 1989. Women, substance abuse and self-help. In *Drugs and British society*, S. McGregor (ed.), 101–15. London: Routledge.
Ettorre, E. 1992. *Women and substance use*. London: Macmillan.
Faccioli, P. & E. Quargnolo 1987. Il principe troppo azzurro. Una ricerca sui tossicodipendenti. *Dei Delitti e delle Pene* **5**, 1, 25–53.
Facy, F., E. Le Huede, H. Ramirez 1991. Drug addicts and syringe sharing in France: epidemiological study 1988. *International Journal of the Addictions* **26**, 5, 515–29.
Facy, F., D. Rosch, P. Angel, D. Touzeau, J-P. Cordonnier, F. Petit 1991. Drug addicts attending specialised institutions: towards a drug addiction data bank?. *Drug and Alcohol Dependence* **27**, 9, 43–50.
Falcone, G. 1991. *Cose di Cosa Nostra*. Milano: Rizzoli.
Fehervary, J. 1989. Drug policy in Austria. See Albrecht & van Kalmthout (1989), 63–88.
Feldman, H. 1968. Ideological supports to becoming and remaining a heroin addict. *Journal of Health and Social Behaviour.* **9**, 131–9.
Field, F. 1989. *Losing out: the emergence of Britain's underclass*. Oxford: Blackwell.
Fijnault, C. 1990. Organized crime: a comparison between the United States of America and Western Europe. *British Journal of Criminology* **30**, 321–40.
Finestone, H. 1957. Cats, kicks and colour. *Social Problems* **5**, 1.
Fish, D. 1962. *Airline detective*. London: Collins.
Fleming, P. (ed.) 1990. *The years ahead*. Winchester: Wessex Regional Health Authority.
Fleming, P., M. Poling, A. Feltham 1992. Drug services in the USSR. *International Journal on Drug Policy* **3**, 1, 28–30.
Flood, S. 1991. *Illicit drugs and organized crime: issues for a unified Europe*. Chicago: Office of International Criminal Justice.
Flosi, L. 1988. La dimensione internazionale della criminalita' organizzata. In *Forme di organizzazione criminale e terrorismo*, F. Ferracuti (ed.). Milano: Giuffre'.
Follett, et al. 1986. HTLV-III antibody in drug abusers in the west of Scotland: the Edinburgh connection. *The Lancet* **1**, 446.
Forsyth, A., R. Hammersley, T. Lavelle, K. Murray 1992. Geographical aspects of

scoring illegal drugs. *British Journal of Criminology* **32**, 3, 292–309.

Foster, J. 1990. *Villains*. London: Routledge.

Fountain, N. 1988. *Underground: the London alternative press 1966–74*. London: Comedia-Routledge.

Fraser, A. & M. George 1988. Changing trends in drug use: an initial follow-up of a local heroin using community. *British Journal of Addiction* **84**, 655–63.

Frith, S. 1978. *The sociology of rock*. London: Constable.

Frith, S. & H. Horne 1987. *Art into pop*. London: Methuen.

Funes, J & O. Romani 1985. *Dejar la heroina*. Madrid: Cruz Roja Espanola/ Direccion General de Accion Social.

Galante, G. 1986. Cent'anni di mafia. In *L'immaginario mafioso*, G. Galante (ed.). Bari: Dedalo.

Gallino, L. 1978. *Dizionario di Sociologia*. Torino: UTET.

Gallo, E. & V. Ruggiero 1985. Il crimine presunto e il delinquente-lavoratore. *Primo Maggio* 23/24, 46–71.

Gallo, E., V. Ruggiero, R. Silvi 1980. *Gli ostelli dello sciamano: alle radici della tosssicodipendenza e del controllo istituzionale*. Milano: Tranchida.

Gambetta, D. 1992. *La mafia Siciliana: un'industria della protezione privata*. Torino: Einaudi.

Gerkin, D., L. Judd, S. Rovner 1977. Career dynamics of female heroin addicts. *American Journal of Drug and Alcohol Abuse* **6**, 1–23.

Gerlach, R. & W. Schneider 1992. Acceptance and abstinence? *International Journal on Drug Policy* **3**, 2, 83–6.

Ghodse, H. 1983. Treatment of drug addiction in London. *The Lancet*, 19 March.

Giggs, J. 1991. The epidemiology of contemporary drug abuse. See Whynes & Bean (1991), 145–75.

Glass, M. 1982. *The dependence phenomenon*. Massachussets: MIT.

Goldstein, P., D. Lipton, E. Preble, I. Sobel, T. Miller, W. Abbott, W. Paige, F. Soto 1984. The marketing of street heroin in New York city. *Journal of Drug Issues* **3**, 553–66.

Gordon, A. M. 1973. Patterns of delinquency in drug addiction. *British Journal of Psychiatry* **122**, 205–10.

——1983. Drugs and delinquency: a ten year follow-up of drug clinic patients. *British Journal of Psychiatry* **142**, 169–73.

Gossop, M. & M. Grant (eds) 1990. *Preventing and controlling drug abuse*. Geneva: World Health Organisation.

Gould, A. 1989. Cleaning the people's home: recent developments in Sweden's addiction policy. *British Journal of Addiction* **84**, 731–41.

——1990. Alcohol and drug policies in Sweden and the UK: a study of two countries. In *Social Policy Review 1989–90*, N. Manning & C. Ungerson (eds), 229–50. Harlow: Longman.

Gouldner, W. 1970. *The coming crisis of western sociology*. London: Heinemann.

Green, J. 1988. *Days in the life: voices from the English underground 1961–71*. London: Heinemann-Minerva.

Green, P. 1991. *Drug couriers*. London: The Howard League for Penal Reform.

Greenberg, D. F. 1990. The cost-benefit of imprisonment. *Social Justice* **17**, 4, 49–75.

Grieve, J. 1993. Thinking the "unthinkable". *Criminal Justice Matters* **12**, 8.

Grob, P. 1993. The needle park in Zurich. *European Journal on Criminal Policy and Research*, **1**, 2, 48–60.

Grosso, L. 1992. Piu' alcool che coca per chi usa eroina. *ASPE* **11**, 15, 16.

Gruppo, Abele. 1992. *Le citta' europee e la droga*. Torino: Edizioni Gruppo Abele.

Guardian 25 April 1990: Train gangs turned to drugs.

——11 October 1990. Drugs flood into Britain from Europe.

Hall, S. & T. Jefferson (eds) 1976. *Resistance through rituals: subcultures in postwar Britain*. London: Hutchinson.

Hamid, A. 1990. The political economy of crack related violence. *Contemporary Drug Problems* Spring, 31–78.

Hammersley, R., A. Forsyth, V. Morrison, J. Davies 1989. The relationship between crime and opioid use. *British Journal of Addictions* **84**, 1029–43.

Hammersley, R., A. Forsyth, T. Lavelle 1990. The criminality of new drug users in Glasgow. *British Journal of Addictions* **85**, 1583–94.

Hanson, B., G. Beschner, J.M. Walters, E. Bovelle 1985. *Life with heroin: voices from the inner city*. Lexington: Lexington Books.

Hartnoll, R. 1986. Current situation relating to drug abuse assessment in European countries. *Bulletin on Narcotics* **38**, 1/2, 65–80.

——1989. The international context. In *Drugs and British society*, S. MacGregor (ed.), 36–51. London: Routledge.

Hartnoll, R., U. Avico, F. Ingold, K. Lange, L. Lenke, A. O'Hare, A. de Roij-Motshagen 1989. A multi-city study of drug misuse in Europe. *Bulletin on Narcotics* **XLI**, 1/2, 3–27.

Hartnoll, R. & M. C. Mitcheson et al. 1980. Evaluation of heroin maintenance in controlled trial. *Archives of General Psychiatry* **37**, 877–84.

Haw, S. 1985. *Drug problems in Greater Glasgow*. Glasgow: Standing Conference on Drug Abuse.

Hebenton, B. & T. Thomas 1992. Rocky path to Europol. *Druglink* November/December, 8–10.

Hedrich, D. 1990. Prostitution and AIDS risks among female drug users in Frankfurt. In *AIDS, Drugs and Prostitution*, M. Plant (ed.), 159–74. London: Routledge.

Heidensohn, F. & M. Farrell (eds) 1991. *Crime in Europe*. London: Routledge

Held, D. & J. B. Thompson, (eds) (1989), *Social theory of modern societies: Anthony Giddens and his critics*, Cambridge: Cambridge University Press.

Helmer, J. 1975. *Drugs and minority oppression*, New York: Seabury Press.

Henman, A. 1985. Cocaine futures. See A. Henman et al., (eds) (1985), 118–89.

Henman, A., R. Lewis, A. Malyon (eds) 1985. *Big deal: the politics of the illicit drug business*. London: Pluto Press.

Henry, S. 1978. *The hidden economy: the context and control of borderline crime*. London: Martin Robertson.

Hobbs, D. 1988. *Doing the business*. Oxford: Oxford University Press.

——1993. *The craft of crime: interviews with three professional criminals*. London: BBC Radio Four programme, August.

——1994. Professional and organized crime in Britain. In *The Oxford handbook of criminology*, M. Maguire, R. Morgan, R. Reiner (eds), 441–68. Oxford: Oxford University Press.

Home Office 1990. *Criminal statistics, England and Wales 1989*. London: HMSO.

Hope, T. & M. Shaw (eds) 1988. *Communities and crime reduction*. London: HMSO.

Hopkinson, N. 1991. *Fighting drugs trafficking in the Americas and Europe*. Wilton Park Papers 43. London: HMSO.

Hughes, P. 1977. *Behind the wall of respect: community experiments in heroin addiction control*. Chicago: University of Chicago Press.

Hughes, P., G. A. Crawford, N. Barker, S. Shumann, J. H. Jaffe 1971. The social structure of a heroin copping community. *American Journal of Psychiatry* **128**, 5, 43–50.

Hunt, L. & C. Chambers 1976. *The heroin epidemics: a study of heroin use in the United States 1965–1975*. New York: Spectrum Books.

Hyder, K. 1993. Brand name boasts of drug dealers. *Evening Standard*, 4 October, 20.

Il Manifesto, 7 November 1979: Eroina.

Inciardi, J. A. 1986. *The war on drugs: heroin, cocaine, crime, and public policy*. Palo Alto, CA: Mayfield.

Inciardi, J. 1987. Drug abuse in the Georgian SSR. *Journal of Psychoactive Drugs* **19**, 4, 329–34.

Inciardi, J. (ed.) 1991. *The drug legalization debate*. Newbury Park, Ca.: Sage.

Inciardi, J. & D. McBride 1989. Legalisation: a high risk alternative in the war on drugs. *American Behavioural Scientist* **32**, 259–89.

Independent, The, 25 April 1990. Drug link to Great Train Robber's murder.

Inglis, B. 1976. *The opium war*. London: Coronet.

Ingold, F. 1985a. Heroin users and economic dependence, *International Criminal Police Review*, **391**, 208–13.

——1985b. Le processus de la dependence chez les heroinomanes. *Annales Medico-Psychologiques* **143**, 63, 585–93.

——1986. Study of deaths related to drug abuse in France and Europe. *Bulletin on Narcotics* **38**, 1/2, 81–9.

Ingold, F. & S. Ingold 1986. The imprisonment of drug addicts and the process of dependence. See Community Epidemiology Work Group (1986).

——1989. The effects of liberalization of syringe sales on the behaviour of intravenous drug users in France. *Bulletin on Narcotics* **XLI**, 1/2, 67–72.

Ingold, F., S. Ingold, S. Brammoville, C. Vaidis 1986. *Le toxicomanes incarcérés*. Paris: IREP.

Ingold, F., M. Madianos, D. Madianou, B. Brigos, J. Anto, J. Cami, C. James, N. Dorn, N. South 1988. *Drugs, alcohol and multiple deprivation: a pilot study in Athens, Barcelona and London*. mimeo, Paris: IREP (Institut de Recherche en Epidemiologie de la Pharmacodependance).

Ingold, F. & C. Olivenstein 1983. Preliminary findings of an epidemiological survey of drug addiction in Paris. *Bulletin on Narcotics* **35**, 3, 73–9.

ILPS (Inner London Probation Service) 1990. *A prison within a prison: a study of foreign prisoners*. London: ILPS.

Insolera, G. & L. Stortoni 1976. Un'altra legge speciale: la legge sulla droga. *La Questione Criminale* **2**, 1, 28–41.

International Journal on Drug Policy 1992a. Special issue focussing on Rotterdam, as site for Fourth International Conference on Reduction of Drug Related Harm.

International Journal on Drug Policy **3**, 4.

——1992b. Injecting drug use identified in 73 different countries: drug injecting now occurs on a global scale and increasing rapidly in Russia and Eastern Europe. *International Journal on Drug Policy* **3**, 3, 117.

——1992c. Radioactive pot and opium poppies found at Chernobyl. *International Journal on Drug Policy* **3**, 64.

INCB 1987. *Annual report.* New York: International Narcotics Control Board.

Interpol 1990. The drugs situation in Europe after 1992. *International Criminal Police Review* **425**, 2532.

ISDD 1991. *Drug misuse in Britain.* London: Institute for the Study of Drug Dependence.

ISDD/M. Ashton (eds) 1993. *National audit of drug misuse in Britain 1992.* London: Institute for the Study of Drug Dependence.

James, I. P. & P. T. D'Orban 1970. Patterns of delinquency among British heroin addicts. *Bulletin of Narcotics* **22**, 13–19.

Jansen, A. 1991. *Cannabis in Amsterdam: a geography of hashish and marijuana.* Netherlands: Mulderberg.

Jarvis, G. & H. Parker 1989. Young heroin users and crime. *British Journal of Criminology* **29**, 2, 175–85.

Jenner, H. 1986. Sweden. See LABOS (1986).

Jennings, A., P. Lashmar, V. Simson 1990. *Scotland Yard's cocaine connection.* London: Jonathon Cape.

Jepsen, J. 1989. Drug policies in Denmark. See Albrecht & van Kalmthout (1989), 107–42.

Jervis, G. 1976. L'ideologia della droga. *Quaderni Piacentini* 58/59, 39–52.

Jessop, B., H. Kastendiek, K. Nielson, O. Pedersen (eds) 1991. *The politics of flexibility.* Aldershot: Edward Elgar.

Johnson, B., P. Goldstein, E. Preble, J. Schmeidler, D. Lipton, B. Spunt, T. Miller 1985. *Taking care of business: the economics of crime by heroin abusers.* Lexington: Lexington Books.

Johnson, B., T. Williams, K. Dei, H. Sanabria 1990. Drug abuse in the inner city: impact on hard drug users and the community. In *Drugs and Crime*, M. Tonry & J.Q. Wilson (eds). Chicago: University of Chicago Press.

Jones, S. & R. Power 1990. Observation to intervention: drug trends in west London. *International Journal on Drug Policy* **2**, 1, 13–15.

Kaiser, G. 1985. *Criminologia.* Milano: Giuffre'.

Kala, M. & T. Borkowski 1990. Drug addiction in Poland and criminalistic traces. *Forensic Science International* **46**, 129–32.

Kaletsky, A. 1993. Crack down on guns and you crack down on crack. *Sunday Telegraph*, 24 October.

Kaplan, C. et al. 1985. Cocaine and socio-cultural groups in the Netherlands. *Epidemiology of Drug Abuse: Research, Clinical and Social Perspectives* IV, 5–16. Rockville: NIDA.

Kaplan, C., M. Morival, C. Sterk 1986. Needle-exchange IV drug users and street IV drug users: a comparison of background characteristics, needle and sex practices, and AIDS attitudes. See *Community Epidemiology Working Group* (1986), iv-16–24.

Kendall, R. 1991. The rôle of Interpol in the control of cocaine trafficking. See Bruno (1991), 397–8.

——1993. Cited in *The Observer*, 28 November, 1.

Klingemann, H. 1991. The motivation for change from problem alcohol and heroin use. *British Journal of Addiction* **86**, 727–44.

Kohn, M. 1992. *Dope girls: the birth of the British drug underground*. London: Lawrence & Wishart.

Kokkevi, A. 1986. Greece. See LABOS (1986).

Korf, D. 1987. Eind van een liijn?. *Intermediair* **24**, 9.

——1990. Cannabis retail markets in Amsterdam. *International Journal on Drug Policy* **2**, 1, 23–7.

Kreuzer, A., R. Romer-Klees, K-H. Dufner 1991a. Perspectives on drug users. In *Police research in the Federal Republic of Germany*, E. Kube & H. Storzer (eds) 151–62. Berlin: Springer.

Kreuzer, A., R. Romer-Klees, H. Schneider 1991b. *Beschaffungskriminalitat Drogenabhangiger*. Wiesbaden.

La Repubblica 1990. L'eroina e' cosa nostra. 23 February.

——Spaccio di eroina. Quattordici carabinieri rinviati a giudizio. 22 March.

——A giudizio 19 persone. Eroina dietro le sbarre, ci pensava il secondino. 8 May.

——Blitz nella notte contro i narcos. Scoperta una baita-laboratorio in mezzo al bosco. 23 May.

——Potevano sfornare quintali di droga. 24 May.

La Stampa 16 June 1989. Arrestata una guardia carceraria sospettata di procurare eroina ai detenuti delle Vallette.

——28 March 1990. Nordafricani manovali dell'eroina.

——6 May 1990. Rapivano bambini per non fallire.

——18 May 1990. La polizia si ribella alle sentenze miti.

LABOS (Workshop for social policy studies) 1986. *European Report on Drug Dependency Services: Users, Practitioners and Organizational Features in Individual European Situations*. Rome: LABOS.

Labrousse, A. 1991. *La drogue, l'argent et les armes*. Paris: Fayard.

Lart, R. 1992. British medical perception from Rolleston to Brain: changing images of the addict and addiction. *International Journal on Drug Policy* **3**, 118–25.

Lavelle, T., R. Hammersley, A. Forsyth, D. Bain 1991. The use of Buprenorphine and Temazepam by drug injectors. *Journal of Addictive Diseases* **10**(3), 5–14.

Lee, R. 1992. Dynamics of the Soviet illicit drug market. *Crime, Law and Social Change* **17**, 3, 177–234.

Leech, K. 1991. The junkies' doctors and the London drug scene in the 1960s: some remembered fragments. In *Policing & prescribing: the British system of drug control*, D. K. Whynes & P. Bean (eds), 35–59. London: Macmillan.

LeGendre, B. 1990. Drugs in all their conditions. *International Journal on Drug Policy*, **1**(4), 24–5.

Leigh, D. 1985. *High time*. London: Unwin.

Leroy, B. 1991. *The community of twelve and the drug demand: comparative study of legislations and judicial practice*. Luxembourg: Commission of the European Community.

Letkenmann, P. 1973. *Crime as work*. Englewood Cliffs, NJ: Prentice Hall.

Levai, M. 1991. Drug abuse and trafficking. *Criminal Justice Matters* 6, summer, 4.

Lewis, R. 1989. European markets in cocaine. *Contemporary Crises* 13, 35–52.

——1994. Flexible hierarchies and dynamic disorder: the trading and distribution of illicit heroin in Britain and Europe. In *Heroin addiction and drug policy: the British system*, J. Strang & M. Gossop (eds). Oxford: Oxford University Press.

Lewis, R., R. Hartnoll, S. Bryer, E. Daviaud, M. Mitcheson 1985. Scoring smack: the illicit heroin market in London 1980–83. *British Journal of Addiction* 80, 281–90.

Lindesmith, A. 1965. *The addict and the law*. New York: Vintage Books.

Lindgren, S-A. 1992. A criticism of Swedish drug policy. *International Journal on Drug Policy* 3, 2, 99–104.

Lipiay, G. 1992. Emerging drug problems in Hungary. *International Journal on Drug Policy* 3, 2, 71–5.

Loimer, N. 1992. Opiate use and abuse in Austria. *International Journal on Drug Policy* 3, 2, 87–90.

Loveday, B. 1992. *Contemporary problems of law and order in England and Wales*, Occasional Paper, Institute of Public Policy and Management, University of Central England.

Luckett, C. 1991. Santé: connaitre les consommateurs. In *Geopolitique de la Drogue*, G. Delbrel (ed.). Paris: La Decouverte.

Lundborg, H. & M. Wikman 1986. Drug policy in Sweden. See *Community Epidemiology Working Group* (1986) iv-26–33.

MacGregor, S. (ed.) 1989. *Drugs and British society*. London: Routledge.

Mack, J. 1964. Full-time miscreants, delinquent neighbourhoods and criminal networks. *British Journal of Sociology* XV, 38–53.

Mack, J. & H. Kerner 1975. *The crime industry*. Lexington, Mass.: Lexington & Saxon House.

Madianou, D. et al. 1987. Preliminary results of two nation-wide epidemiological studies of drug use in Greece: a study of known cases and a general population survey. *Bulletin on Narcotics* 39, 69–79.

Magistratura Democratica 1980. *Dossier droga. I processi per droga a Torino dal 1976 al 1980*. Torino: Book Store/Magistratura Democratica.

Manou, D. 1992. *Histories of drug use: case studies of the residents in a drug treatment and rehabilitation unit in Greece*. MA Dissertation, Department of Sociology, University of Essex.

Marozzi, F. & I. Merzagora 1992. Cocaina, una droga sensibile al contesto sociale. *ASPE* 11, 15, 12–13.

Mars, G. 1982. *Cheats at work: an anthropology of work place crime*. London: Allen & Unwin.

McCarthy, T. & T. Kirby 1990. Nigeria heroin link expands Golden Triangle. *The Independent*, 24 July.

McIntosh, M. 1971. Changes in the organization of thieving. In *Images of deviance*, S. Cohen (ed.), 98–133. Harmondsworth: Penguin.

——1975. *The organisation of crime*. London: Macmillan.

McKeganey, N. & F. Boddy 1987. *Drug abuse in Glasgow: an interim report of an exploratory study*. Glasgow: Department of Child Health and Obstetrics, University of Glasgow.

McLaughlin, E. 1992. The democratic deficit: European union and the accountability of the British police. *British Journal of Criminology* **32**, 4, 473–87.

McRobbie, A. 1980. Settling accounts with subcultures: a feminist critique. *Screen Education* **34**, 37–50.

Merlo, G. 1988. La situazione delle tossicodipendenze a Torino. *Salute e Prevenzione* **1**, 15–26.

Merton, R. 1968. *Social theory and social structure*. New York: Free Press.

Miles, R. 1993. *Ruffling feathers: is drug enforcement for the birds?* MA Research Dissertation, Department of Sociology, University of Essex.

Mirza, H., G. Pearson, S. Phillips 1991. *Drugs, people and services in Lewisham: final report of the drug information project*. London: Goldsmiths College, University of London.

Mol, R. & F. Trautmann 1991. The liberal image of the Dutch drug policy. *International Journal on Drug Policy* **2**, 5, 16–21.

Monitoring Research Group 1988. *Injecting equipment exchange schemes: final report*. London: Goldsmiths College, University of London.

Morales, E. 1989. *Cocaine: white gold rush in Peru*. Tucson: University of Arizona Press.

Morrison, V. 1988. Drug misuse and concern about HIV infection in Edinburgh: an interim report. In *Drug questions 4: annual research register*, N. Dorn, L. Lucas, N. South (eds). London: Institute for the Study of Drug Dependence.

——1989. Psychoactive substance use and related behaviours of 135 regular illicit drug users in Scotland. *Drug and Alcohol Dependence* **23**, 2, 95–101.

——1991. Licit and illicit drug initiations and alcohol-related problems amongst illicit drug users in Edinburgh. *Drug and Alcohol Dependence* **27**, 19–27.

——1992. Responding in a crisis: perspectives on HIV, drugs and women's needs from Edinburgh. In *AIDS: Women, drugs and social care*, N. Dorn, S. Henderson & N. South (eds), 30–50. London: Falmer.

Mott, J. 1991. Crime and heroin use. See Whynes & Bean (1991), 77–94.

——(ed.) 1992. *Crack and cocaine in England and Wales*. Home Office Research and Planning Unit Paper 70. London: HMSO.

Murji, K. 1993. Drug enforcement strategies. *The Howard Journal of Criminal Justice* **32**, 3: 215–30.

Musto, D. 1973. *The American disease: origins of narcotic control*. New Haven: Yale University Press.

NACRO 1991. *Prisons, HIV and AIDS*. London: National Association for the Care and Resettlement of Offenders.

Nadelman, E. 1988. The case for legalization. *The Public Interest* **92**, 3–31.

——1989. Drug prohibition in the United States: costs, consequences and alternatives. *Science* **245**, 939–47.

——1990. The DEA in Europe: drug enforcement in comparative and international perspective. working paper. Woodrow Wilson School of Public and International Affairs, Princeton University.

——1993. Should we legalize drugs? Yes. *American Heritage* February/March, 41–8.

NAPO 1990. *Drug users and custody*. London: National Association of Probation Officers.

NDIU 1989. *Drug seizure statistics 1989*. London: National Drugs Intelligence Unit,

New ScotlandYard.

Nelson, D. & P. Victor 1993. Crack in the thin blue line. *The Observer*, 24 October, 23.

Nove, P. 1991. Underground banking systems. *International Criminal Police Review* **431**, 5–9.

O'Brian, L. 1989. Young people and drugs. In *Drugs and British Society*, S. McGregor (ed.), 64–76. London: Routledge.

O'Hare, P., R. Newcombe, A. Matthews, E. Buning, E. Drucker (eds) 1992. *The reduction of drug related harm*. London: Routledge.

O'Kelly, F., G. Bury, B. Cullen, G. Dean 1988. The rise and fall of heroin use in an inner city area of Dublin. *Irish Journal of Medical Science* **157**, 2, 35–8.

Paci, M. 1982. *La struttura sociale italiana*. Bologna: Il Mulino.

Padilla, F. M. 1992. *The gang as an American enterprise*. New Brunswick, NJ: Rutgers University Press.

Palermo, C. 1983. Le forme nuove del crimine organizzato. *Democrazia e Diritto* 23/24, 31–40.

Pantaleone, M. 1966. *Mafia e politica*. Torino: Einaudi.

——1979. *Mafia e droga*. Torino: Einaudi.

Parsinnen, T. 1983 *Secret passions, secret remedies: narcotic drugs in British society, 1820–1930*. Manchester: Manchester University Press.

Pearson, G. 1987a. *The new heroin users*. Oxford: Basil Blackwell.

——1987b. Social deprivation, unemployment and patterns of heroin use. In *A land fit for heroin?*, N. Dorn & N. South (eds), 62–94. London: Macmillan.

——1990. The French connection. *International Journal on Drug Policy* **1**(4), 24–5.

——1991. Drug control policies in Britain. In *Crime and justice: a review of research*, *14*, M. Tonry & N. Morris (eds), 167–227. Chicago: University of Chicago.

——1992. Drugs and criminal justice: a harm reduction perspective. See O'Hare et al. (1992), 15–29.

Pearson, G. & M. Gilman 1994. Local and regional variations in drug misuse: the British heroin epidemic of the 1980s. In *Heroin addiction and drug policy: the British system*, J. Strang & M. Gossop (eds), 102–120. Oxford: Oxford University Press.

Pearson, G., M. Gilman, S. McIver 1987. *Young people and heroin*. Aldershot: Avebury.

Peck, D. & M. Plant 1986. Unemployment and illegal drug use: concordant evidence from a prospective study and from national trends. *British Medical Journal* **293**, 929–31.

Perry, L. 1979. Women and drug use: an unfeminine dependency. London: ISDD.

Picotti, L. 1979. Ricerca nell'area veneta sull'applicazione della legge N. 685. *La Questione Criminale* **5**, 2, 186–201.

Pisapia, G. 1991. Dalla modica quantita' alla modica punibilità. In *Legalizzare la droga. Una ragionevole proposta di sperimentazione*, L. Manconi (ed.). Milano: Feltrinelli.

Pizzorno, A. & P. Arlacchi 1985. *Camorra, contrabbando e mercato della droga in Campania*. Roma: Commissione Parlamentare sul Fenomeno della Mafia.

Platt, J. 1993. Case studies: their uses and limits. *Sociology Review*, February, 8–12.

Police Review 1989. Swiss drugs experiment leads to rise in crime. *Police Review* 18 August, 1656.

Ponti, G.L. 1980. *Compendio di criminologia*. Milano: Cortina.

Porter, R. & V. Elliott 1993. Childish minds in thugs bodies. *Sunday Telegraph*, 24 October, 17.

Power, R. 1987. Smack and pool. *New Society*, 3 July.

——1989. Drugs and the media: prevention campaigns and television. In *Drugs and British society*, S. McGregor (ed.), 129–42. London: Routledge.

Prather, J. & L. S. Fidell 1978. Drug use and abuse among women: an overview. *International Journal of Addiction* **13**, 863–85.

Preble, E. & J. Casey 1969. Taking care of business: the heroin user's life on the street. *The International Journal of the Addictions* **4**, 1, 1–24.

Price, B. 1991. Cocaine trafficking in the United Kingdom. See Bruno (1991), 393–6.

PRT 1991. *The Woolf report: a summary of the main findings and recommendations of the inquiry into prison disturbances*. London: Prison Reform Trust.

Pritchard, M. & E. Laxton 1978. *Busted! The sensational life story of an undercover cop*. London: Mirror Books.

Radio Flash and Radio Torino Popolare 1989. *Vita in Polvere. L'eroina a Torino; storie e iniziative*. Torino: Radio Flash and Radio Torino Popolare.

Ray, O. 1978. *Drugs, society and human behavior*. Saint Louis: Mosby Press.

Raymond, F. 1975. A sociological view of narcotics addiction. *Crime and Delinquency* **21**, 1, 11–18.

Rebelles 1991. Toxicomanie, des chiffres contre une mythologie. *Rebelles* December, 18–20.

Redhead, S. 1993. *Rave off: politics and deviance in contemporary youth culture*. Aldershot: Avebury.

Redlinger, L. 1975. Marketing and distributing heroin: some sociological observations. *Journal of Psychedelic Drugs* **7**, 4, 331–53.

Regione Piemonte 1985. *Relazione sanitaria*. Torino: Servizi Tossicodipendenze.

Reuter, P. 1984. *Disorganized crime: illegal markets and the Mafia*. Cambridge, Mass.:MIT Press.

Reuter, P., R. MacCoun, P. Murphy 1990. *Money from crime: a study of the economics of drug dealing in Washington D.C.*. Santa Monica, CA: RAND Corporation.

Ribeiro, N. 1986. Portugal. See LABOS (1986).

Richardson, C. 1991. *My manor: the autobiography of Charlie Richardson*. London: Sidgwick & Jackson.

Ricolfi, L., S. Scaramuzzi, L. Sciolla 1988. *Essere giovani a Torino*. Torino: Rosenberg & Sellier.

Rinascita. 1984. Una barriera da abbattere. *Geografia della dipendenza*. 10 February.

Robertson, J., A. Bucknall, P. Welsby, J. Roberts, J. Inglis, J. Peutherer, R. Brettle 1986. Epidemic of AIDS related virus (HTLV III/LAV) infection among intravenous drug abusers. *British Medical Journal* **292**, 527–9.

Rolli, A. 1985. Il problema eroina oggi. In *Droga: femminile plurale*, Garelli, A. M. (ed.). Torino: Gruppo Abele.

Rosenbaum, M. 1981. Sex rôles among deviants: the woman addict. *International Journal of Addiction* **16**, 859–77.

——1982. *Women on heroin*. New Brunswick, NJ: Rutgers University Press.

Rosenbaum, M. & S. Murphy 1990. Women and addiction: process, treatment and outcome. In *The collection and interpretation of data from hidden populations*, E.Y. Lambert (ed.), 120–27. Rockville, MD: National Institute on Drug Abuse.

Royal College of Psychiatrists 1987. *Drug scenes*. London: Gaskell.

Ruggiero, V. 1986. La droga come merce. *Criminologia* **6**, 22–8.

——1987. Turin today: premodern society or postindustrial bazaar?. *Capital and Class* **31**, 25–38.

——1992. *La roba: economie e culture dell'eroina*. Parma: Pratiche Editrice.

——1993a. Brixton, London: a drug culture without a drug economy? *International Journal of Drug Policy* **4**, 2, 83–90.

——1993b. *Perceptions of the drug phenomenon in central Lambeth*. London: Lambeth Drugs Prevention Team/Home Office.

——1993c. Organised crime in Italy: testing alternative definitions. *Social & Legal Studies*, **2**, 2, 131–48.

——1993d. The Camorra: "clean" capital and organised crime. In *Global crime connections*, F. Pearce & M. Woodiwiss (eds), 141–61. London: Macmillan.

——1994. Organised crime and drug economies. *International Journal of Drug Policy* **5**, 2, 106–114.

Ruggiero, V. & A. Vass 1992. Heroin use and the formal economy. *British Journal of Criminology* **32**, 3, 273–91.

Rusconi, M. & G. Blumir 1978. *La droga e il sistema*. Milano: Feltrinelli.

Sabourin, S. 1991. Drug money. *International Criminal Police Review* **431**, 2–5.

Samson, R. 1990. Perspectives for the development of drug misuse policies as seen from the Netherlands. In *The years ahead*, P. Fleming (ed.), 25–46. Winchester: Wessex Regional Health Authority.

Savona, E., N. Dorn, T. Ellis 1994. *Cocaine markets and law enforcement*. Rome: UNICRI.

Scheerer, S. 1989. Killing the ill? Heroin and AIDS in West Germany. See Albrecht & van Kalmthout (1989), 161–74.

Scheerer, S. & I. Vogt 1989. *Drogen und drogenpolitik*. Frankfurt/New York: Campus.

Schultz, H. 1989. Drugs and drug politics in Switzerland. See Albrecht & van Kalmthout (1989), 361–80.

Schur, E. 1964. Drug addiction under British policy. In *The other side*, H. Becker (ed.). New York: Free Press.

Sciacchitano, G. 1991. Possible co-operation between Italy and the Andean countries in substituting coca plantations and repressing drug trafficking. See Bruno (1991), 219–22.

Scraton, P. & N. South 1984. The ideological construction of the hidden economy: private justice and work-related crime. *Contemporary Crises* **8**, 1, 1–18.

Scott, P. & J. Marshall 1991. *Cocaine politics: drugs, armies, and the CIA in Central America*. Berkeley: University of California Press.

Sellal, P. 1991. International cocaine traffic in France and the part played by South American nationals. See Bruno, F (1991), 415–19.

Serfaty, A. 1990. HIV infection and drug use in France: an overview of the epidemic and public health and public health strategies. In Community Epidemiology Work Group. *Epidemiological trends in drug abuse*, Rockville: NIDA.

Shapiro, H. 1989. *Crack: a briefing*. London: ISDD.

——1991. Contemporary cocaine use in Britain. In *Drug misuse in Britain* ISDD,

40–45. London: ISDD.

——1993. Where does all the snow go?. In *Cocaine and crack*, P. Bean (ed.). London: Macmillan.

——1994. Only way – or no way? *Druglink* **9**, 12–15.

Shover, N. 1973. The social organization of burglary. *Social Problems* **20**, 4, 499–514.

Soggiu, P. 1991. Cocaine trafficking in the Mediterranean area. See Bruno (1991), 382–7.

Solans Soteras, M. 1991. Cocaine trafficking in Europe. See Bruno (1991) 390–92.

Solarz, A. 1989. Drug policy in Sweden. See Albrecht & van Kalmthout (1989), 343–60.

South, N. 1988. *Policing for profit: the private security sector*. London: Sage.

——1992. Moving murky money: drug trafficking, law enforcement and the pursuit of criminal profits. In *Offenders and victims: theory and policy*, D. Farrington & S. Walklate (eds), 167–93. London:British Society of Criminology/ISTD.

——1993. Criminal justice versus public health: decriminalisation, legalisation and harm reduction. *Criminal justice matters* **12**, 10.

——1994. Drugs: control, crime and criminological studies. In *The Oxford handbook of criminology*, M. Maguire, R. Morgan, R. Reiner (eds), 393–440. Oxford: Oxford University Press.

——(ed.) 1995a. *Drugs, crime and criminal justice, Vol. 1: histories and use, theories and debates*. Aldershot: Dartmouth.

——(ed.) 1995b. *Drugs, crime and criminal justice, Vol. 2: cultures and markets, crime and criminal justice*. Aldershot: Dartmouth.

Spear, H. B. & J. Mott 1992. A brief history of the control of cocaine in the United Kingdom. In *Crack and cocaine in England and Wales*, J. Mott (ed.), 1–11. London: Home Office Research and Planning Unit Paper 70.

Stewart. T. 1987. *The heroin users*. London: Pandora.

Stewart-Clark, J. 1986. *Report of the committee of inquiry into the drugs problem in the member states of the community*. Strasbourg: European Parliament.

Stimson, G. 1987. The war on heroin: British policy and the international trade in illicit drugs. In *A land fit for heroin?* N. Dorn & N. South (eds), 35–61. London: Macmillan.

——July 1992. Epidemiology of injecting drug use. Paper to Eighth International Conference on AIDS.

Stimson, G. & E. Oppenheimer 1982. *Heroin addiction: Treatment and control in Britain*. London: Tavistock.

Stourton, E. 1993. Will they have to legalise it? *Sunday Telegraph*, 3 October, 22.

Strang, J. & M. Gossop (eds) 1994. *Heroin addiction and drug policy: the British system*. Oxford: Oxford University Press.

Strang, J., P. Griffiths, M. Gossop 1990. Crack and cocaine use in South London drug addicts: 1987–1989. *British Journal of Addictions* **85**, 193–6.

Sutter, A. 1966. The world of the righteous dope-fiend. *Issues in Criminology* **2**, 2, 177–222.

Sutton, M. 1993. From receiving to thieving: the market for stolen goods and the incidence of theft. *Home Office Research Bulletin* **34**, 3–8.

Sutton, M. & A. Maynard 1992. *What is the size and nature of the "drug" problem in the UK?*, YARTIC Occasional Paper 3. Centre for Health Economics, University of York.

Sykes G. & D. Matza 1957. Techniques of neutralization: a theory of delinquency. *American Sociological Review* **22**, 6.

Taylor, A. 1993. *Women drug users*. Oxford: Clarendon Press.

Taylor, I., P. Walton, J. Young 1973. *The new criminology*. London: Routledge.

Taylor, L. 1984. *In the underworld*. London: Unwin.

Thompson H. S. 1972. *Fear and loathing in Las Vegas*. London: Paladin.

Tisdall, S. & E. Vulliamy 1992. Cocaine blitz traps top dealers. *The Guardian*, 29 September.

Tobolska-Rydz, H. 1986. Problems of drug abuse and preventive measures in Poland. *Bulletin on Narcotics* **38**, 1/2, 99–105.

Torrens, M., L. San, J. Peri, J. Olle 1991. Cocaine abuse among heroin addicts in Spain. *Drug and Alcohol Dependence* **27**, 29–34.

Townsend, P. 1987. *Poverty and labour in London*. London: Low Pay Unit.

——1990. Underclass and overclass: the widening gulf between social classes in Britain in the 1980s. In *Sociology in action*, G. Payne & M. Cross (eds). London: Macmillan.

Treaster, J. 1992. Echoes of prohibition: 20 years of war on drugs and no victory yet. *New York Times*, 14 June.

Trebach, A. 1982. *The heroin solution*. New Haven, Conn.: Yale University Press.

Trigilia, C. 1986. Small firm development and political subcultures in Italy. *European Sociological Review* **213**, 161–75.

Trimble, J., C. Bolek, S. Niemcryk 1992. *Ethnic and multicultural drug abuse*. New York: Howarth Press.

Trocchi, A. 1992. *Cain's book*. London: Calder.

Turner, B. 1987. *Medical power and social knowledge*. London: Sage.

Tyler, A. 1986. *Street drugs*. London: New English Library.

Unell, I. 1987. Drugs and deprivation. *Druglink* **2**, 6, 14–15.

Van Duyne, P. & M. Levi 1991. Enterprise crime in the Netherlands and the UK. Paper presented at the British Criminology Conference, York 1991.

van Haastrecht, H., J. van den Hoek, C. Bardoux, A. Leentvaar-Kuypers, R. Coutinho 1991. The course of the HIV epidemic among intravenous drug users in Amsterdam, The Netherlands. *American Journal of Public Health* **81**, 1, 59–62.

Van Vleit, H. 1990. The uneasy decriminalization: a perspective on Dutch drug policy. *Hoftsra Law Review* **18**, 3, 717–50.

Wagstaff, A. & A. Maynard 1988. *Economic aspects of the illicit drug market and drug enforcement policies in the UK*. London: HMSO.

Waldorf, D. 1973. *Careers in dope*. Englewood Cliffs: Prentice-Hall.

Walter, I. 1989. *Secret money: the shadowy world of tax evasion, capital flight and fraud*. London: Unwin.

Watson, P. 1989. Drug use and policy in Poland in the 1980s. *International Journal of Health Services* **19**, 3.

——1991. Supply and demand: lessons from Poland. *Druglink* **6**(4), 12–13.

Wever, L. 1992. Drug policy changes in Europe and the USA: alternatives to international warfare. *International Journal on Drug Policy* **3**, 4, 176–81.

White, P. 1989. An ancient Indian herb turns deadly: Coca. *National Geographic* **175**, 1, 3–47.

WHO 1990. *Sociocultural factors in drug abuse*. Geneva: World Health Organisation.

WHO 1992. *European summary on drug abuse.* Geneva: World Health Organisation.

Whynes, D. K. & P. Bean (eds) 1991. *Policing and prescribing: the British system of drug control.* London: Macmillan.

Wiarda, J. 1989. Drug policies in Western Europe. See Albrecht & van Kalmthout (1989), 29–40.

Wiepert, G. D., P. T. D'Orban, T. H. Bewley 1979. Delinquency by opiate addicts treated at two London clinics. *British Journal of Psychiatry* **134**, 14–23.

Williams, T. 1989. *The cocaine kids: the inside story of a teenage drug ring.* New York: Addison-Wesley.

——1992. *Crack house: notes from the end of the line.* New York: Addison-Wesley.

Willis, P. 1978. *Profane culture.* London: Routledge.

Wilson, J. Q. 1990. Against the legalization of drugs. *Commentary* **89**, 21–28.

Wilson, J. Q. & G. Kelling 1982. Broken windows. *The Atlantic Review*, March, 29–38.

Wisotsky, S. 1986. *Breaking the impasse in the war on drugs.* Westport, Ct.: Greenwood Press.

Worall, A. 1990. *Offending women: female law breakers and the criminal justice system*, London: Routledge.

Young, J. 1971a. *The drugtakers.* London: Paladin.

——1971b. The police as amplifiers of deviancy. In *Images of deviance*, S. Cohen (ed.), 27–61. Harmondsworth: Penguin.

——1987. Deviance. In *The new introducing sociology*, P. Worsley (ed.), 407–450. Harmondsworth: Penguin.

Zinberg, N. 1984. *Drug, set and setting: the basis for controlled intoxicant use.* New Haven, Conn.: Yale University Press.

Zincani, V. 1989. *La criminalita' organizzata: strutture criminali e controllo sociale.* Bologna: Clueb.

Index